THE VITAMIN CURE

for Infant and Toddler Health Problems

RALPH K. CAMPBELL, M.D.
AND ANDREW W. SAUL, PH.D.

Basic Health
PUBLICATIONS, INC.

The information contained in this book is based upon the research and personal and professional experiences of the authors. It is not intended as a substitute for consulting with your physician or other healthcare provider. Any attempt to diagnose and treat an illness should be done under the direction of a healthcare professional.

The publisher does not advocate the use of any particular healthcare protocol but believes the information in this book should be available to the public. The publisher and authors are not responsible for any adverse effects or consequences resulting from the use of the suggestions, preparations, or procedures discussed in this book. Should the reader have any questions concerning the appropriateness of any procedures or preparation mentioned, the authors and the publisher strongly suggest consulting a professional healthcare advisor.

Basic Health Publications, Inc.
28812 Top of the World Drive
Laguna Beach, CA 92651
949-715-7327 • www.basichealthpub.com

Library of Congress Cataloging-in-Publication Data

Campbell, Ralph K.
   The vitamin cure for infant and toddler health problems / Ralph K. Campbell, M.D. and Andrew W. Saul, Ph.D.—First edition.
      pages cm
   Includes bibliographical references and index.
   ISBN 978-1-59120-303-2 (alk. paper)
   1. Orthomolecular therapy. 2. Infants—Diseases—Alternative treatment.
3. Vitamin therapy. I. Saul, Andrew W. II. Title.
   RJ53.V57C362 2013
   615.3'280832—dc23

                                                        2013014489

Editor: Karen Anspach
Typesetting/Book design: Gary A. Rosenberg
Cover design: Mike Stromberg

Printed in the United States of America

10 9 8 7 6 5 4 3 2 1

CONTENTS

To Fred Rogers (1928–2003)

ACKNOWLEDGMENTS

Attitudes develop early in the education process, but much down-to-earth education begins after formal education. Most of what I learned of nutrition and infant care began and continued in both my home and office. My wife, Jan, rode the first wave of rethinking what "real" foods really are. Everyday care of our own infants, and listening to the parents of infants in my practice, proved to provide important post-doctoral education. I am indebted to these educators. In addition I would like to mention some nutrition "greats" who put me on, and kept me on, the right track. They not only imparted their knowledge but encouraged me to tell parents what works: Jack Challem, William G. Crook, Lendon H. Smith, and Andrew W. Saul.

—Ralph K. Campbell, M.D.

I'd like to thank all who have helped me learn to parent. In addition to setting good examples, my parents and brothers taught me much that came in mighty handy later. Drs. Fredrick R. Klenner and Robert F. Cathcart III provided the world with high-dose vitamin C protocols and practical advice that helped me get my children well every time I followed their lead, and that soon became always. I also thank my children for their cooperation. People I have never met face to face have nonetheless reached me through their books, including Drs. Haim G. Ginott, Richard Alpert (aka Ram Dass), Thomas W. Phelan,

Richard Passwater, Lendon H. Smith, and Linus Pauling. My most especial appreciation is reserved for Colleen, my much better half and number-one fan.

—Andrew W. Saul

Both authors would like to very much thank Dr. Atsuo Yanagisawa for writing the foreword to this book. We are also grateful to Dr. Thomas E. Levy and Helen Saul Case for writing two of this book's Appendices.

FOREWORD

Parents bear children, and the children grow up to give birth to the next generation. That is how we humans have built our tree of life for thousands of years, and it is also our duty to continue that line. With that purpose, no one would argue against the importance of a safe environment for children to grow up healthily.

However, this is an era with an abundance of danger for our children's health, like no other time in our long history. Today's children live surrounded by environmental pollution, processed foods soaked in additives, low nutrition, and junk foods. In the last few years in Japan, where I live, serious health concerns have been raised by radioactive contamination from the incident at a nuclear plant in March 2011.

In this unsafe time parents and doctors have to take an important role to protect our children's health. This must be done not only with traditional knowledge, but also with a deeper understanding of the health effects of recent environmental changes. Infants' and small children's health are an especially delicate matter because their organs are in a rapid growth period in which they gain sufficient biological functions. Serious illness can be caused if nutrition intake is unbalanced during this period. The health care profession can be a very difficult practice because of the delicateness and importance of children's health.

Experts of nutritional medicine (and also my dear friends) Dr. Ralph K.Campbell and Dr. Andrew W. Saul have written this inspiring book to help you with the important task of protecting your children's health. Dr. Campbell is highly knowledgeable in nutritional therapy and a very experienced pediatrician. Dr. Saul is a highly recognized expert in nutritional medicine as well as an advocate who spreads meaningful knowledge to the wide population. What they have achieved here is a book with a view focusing on orthomolecular medicine. Orthomolecular medicine describes the practice of preventing and treating disease by providing the body with optimal amounts of substances that are natural to the body. Intake of essential nutrients such as vitamins, minerals, and amino acids from supplements, along with a balanced diet, will prevent and treat illness and lead to ideal health for infants and small children.

Everybody knows that "you are what you eat." Newborns grow up on breast milk or whatever else they eat. Their health depends on the amount and balance of nutrients in these "foods." When a child gets sick, the first choice for a cure is not to give drugs, but to treat with the right nutrition. Vitamins especially are known to be more effective at times in treating illness than medicine. Medicine should not be the first choice for treatment except in an urgent situation, because its effects on children is likely to be too strong and cause side effects.

This book should be a bible not only for parents with small children, but also for health care professionals who are practicing or planning to practice nutritional therapy. Children are not just miniature adults, and there must be adequate guidebooks to treat them. I strongly believe that this book will provide guidance towards the first-choice nutritional approach, so that many children can live healthier lives and be free of illness and the dangerous side effects of modern medicine.

—Atsuo Yanagisawa, M.D., Ph.D.
President, International Society
for Orthomolecular Medicine

INTRODUCTION

In 1977 I (AWS) was a twenty-two-year-old newly minted father. It goes without saying that I knew nothing and learned fast. When my firstborn came into the world, the delivery staff was so busy with details that they just put my little son on a warming table and left him there. This is literally true; I was right there. The warming table had two heat lamps over it, just like the ones uses at fast-food restaurants to keep your fries hot. My little son looked rather lonely over there. So, thinking there would never be a more opportune time to get acquainted, I went over and took a look at him. He was just over eight pounds, but as I had had no younger siblings, he looked pretty small to me. I held out my hand, and he grabbed my little finger with his. His entire hand could not quite encircle my smallest digit. And how about those tiny fingernails, eh?

And now I am a grandfather. Indeed, this book is written by two grandfathers. That may be good. When my first child was born, I needed most what I lacked most: experience. When I was a first-year teacher, I wanted some gray hair. Well, now I have both. A mixed blessing, perhaps. Experience, it has been said, is what you get from bad decisions. Not necessarily. Good decisions also generate experience, the positive kind. And speaking of experience, I am now going to hand you over to Dr. Campbell, the senior member of our writing team. I will be back later, but he's the expert, and as my father always said, "Talk to the organ grinder, not the monkey." Enjoy the book, and enjoy your bambino!

—Andrew W. Saul

CHAPTER 1

HOW I BECAME A PARENT AND A PEDIATRICIAN

During World War II, I (RKC) was fortunate enough to have my older sister live with our family while her husband was in flight training at an airbase that had no accommodations for wives. She was in her last weeks of pregnancy and I was in high school. After the blessed event of her delivering a "perfect" boy, I sometimes played the surrogate father. Breast-feeding, strangely, was not in vogue, but sometimes being a designated bottle-feeder for my little nephew made me feel useful. I learned as just a kid, then, that there was more to feeding than filling a tummy; more to diaper changing than the mundane task—it made him more comfortable. Then and there, pediatrics became my chosen field of medicine.

An eighteen-month stint as a peacetime (barely) Navy Hospital Corpsman helped me rule out other medical careers. I spent much of my service time curing the effects of bad choices while I was practically in charge of what amounted to a venereal disease clinic, and later when I acted as a psychiatrist on a rather "open ward" for the Marines. The GI Bill helped tremendously in furthering my premedical and medical education. The financial aid allowed me to marry my high school sweetheart and for us to produce two marvelous (of course) children, while still in medical school—my first "hands-on" pediatric experience.

Pomona College in Claremont, California, medical school (Yale University) and pediatric residency (Los Angeles Children's Hospital) equipped me as best as a formal education could, leading to the *real* education that a pediatric practice created. It didn't take me long to realize that a standard medical education, including internship and residency training, left much to be desired. The post-war era was perfect for pediatrics. Veterans (consisting of most of the young men of college age) received education benefits. Americans made and exported products worldwide, enabling good wages and ability to achieve the "American Dream." Moms felt respected and seemed content to be full-time mothers. They wanted the "best" care and advice pertaining to the health of their children. Parents learned from us; we learned from the parents. I obtained my fellowship in the American Academy of Pediatrics and enjoyed the effort to keep on top of my chosen specialty through reading and attending meetings. In retrospect, I think my enjoyment began to fade with the advent of medical—so-called "health"—insurance. Insurance providers called the shots as to what procedures and diagnoses would be paid for, or how the physician would be reimbursed for his time and expertise. Lendon Smith signed a book of his that he gave to me, "Ralph, if it isn't fun, don't do it." Insurance providers preferred dealing with the more tangible acute-care things—prescriptions and immunizations—over counseling and diagnosis and treatment of puzzling illnesses. Little by little the fun of being able to share in parents' joy of child rearing and health education diminished.

Cultural changes proceeded at a much slower pace than they do today. Nevertheless, they did proceed, and have been significant: the emphasis on medicines and medical technology as opposed to physician advice on how to achieve good health through self-help education, including nutrition and other lifestyle factors. Processed foods and new environmental toxins slipped into the picture. As the economic boom settled down many mothers entered the job market, pulling them away from home. Add to this the distraction of television geared to hyping up preschoolers, and parenting became more difficult. The result was obvious: Children entering kindergarten were less secure, less prepared to learn.

By 1970, I had reached the end-point of my frustration in being told what I could and could not do in a pediatric practice. Even though I was a well-respected member of pediatric societies in Southern California, I was powerless as I attempted, with others, to even slow the progression of these faulty trends. So, after careful consideration and input from family, we moved my practice from Claremont, California, (air that sometimes should have been declared "unbreathable" was also a factor) to Polson, Montana. I conducted well-child clinics for the Confederated Salish-Kootenai tribes in our county and got the County Health Department stronger by hiring a County Health nurse and other full-time personnel. Later, I established a private pediatric practice. Both the public and the private practices opened my eyes to many new things: deficiencies in care of those who could not afford private care, how private care insurance carriers restricted necessary care and pushed immunizations while not allowing parental input, and widespread ignorance about environmental toxins—or if not ignorance, misinformation disseminated by federal agencies to cover up and help the involved industries. Acting as the county jail doctor for eight years was a real eye-opener. So many inmates were having side effects to medicines they were taking and had no idea of what the drugs were expected to do. Nutrition knowledge was totally absent. My more leisurely pace, ironically, allowed me more time to question the authoritative bodies such as the American Academy of Pediatrics (AAP), the Centers for Disease Control and Prevention (CDC), and the U.S. Environmental Protection Agency (EPA), and do my own research. With the move to Montana, I acquired a cherry orchard. The work complemented my health work by putting me in touch with the EPA and the Department of Agriculture. Developing and marketing a natural fertilizer helped me gain knowledge in plant nutrition, which enhanced my background in human nutrition.

Our local Health Department tried to pass on what I learned to the "busy" practitioners in my county. The more I learned, the more skeptical I became. The more skeptical I became, the lower my ranking as a pediatrician or County Health Officer became. (I often tangled with the State Health Department.) Even while I was Secretary-Treasurer of the Montana Chapter of the AAP (for thirteen years), I battled my colleagues over such things as fluoridation of public water systems, lead screening, sudden infant death (SIDS) prevention, allergies related to attention deficit hyperactivity disorder (ADHD) and middle ear effusion (fluid in the middle ear), and the validity of an ADHD diagnosis itself. Finally, I took a hard look at various immunizations.

At the same time my certainty of the value of megavitamin use, particularly of vitamin C, put me into the outcast category among my peers. These things, plus the Academy's one-sided advocacy on social issues, caused me to drop my emeritus membership status in 2003. In my opinion, this family-oriented, extremely gratifying specialty has disintegrated due to cultural (and pharmaceutical industry) pressures. Almost daily, improper actions of agencies "protecting" us from environmental toxins, food contamination, and harmful drugs and vaccines are exposed. Almost no attention is paid to true preventive measures. Rather, there exists an active disparagement of anything criticizing the practices of these agencies and the producers of pharmaceutical medicines and immunizations. My otherwise seemingly intelligent colleagues are nearly totally ignorant of what constitutes good nutrition or the judicious use of vitamin supplements. They prefer to believe what the uneducated "experts" tell them. I have no intention of throwing in the towel, but it is difficult finding a way to overcome this ignorance and still be "nice."

My situation in thinking about my firstborn was unique. My high school sweetheart and I had patiently (most of the time) waited to marry through my military service and our college years. Then we were whisked from the laid-back Southern California lifestyle to the strange culture of New Haven, Connecticut, and its even stranger medical school ambiance. As one of my wonderfully open Italian classmates put it, our firstborn came "nine months and fifteen minutes after the ceremony." We were home for summer break when the blessed event took place. Ironically, my grandfather, whom I dearly loved, was admitted to the same hospital with a broken hip at the same time. A stroke resulting from surgical manipulation ended in his death on the day my daughter was born—greatly increasing the emotional charge surrounding her birth. One beautiful life enters; another leaves. She was a big, and in my mind, beautiful baby. Actually, she was pretty beat-up, due to a posterior presentation birth. I was so overwhelmed with feelings of gratitude and relief that I truly saw beauty even in her face, though it had been pushed around a bit. Someone, presumably the obstetrician, examined our baby. So somehow, feeling comfortable with the explanation for her bloodied face and other assurances of her being a healthy baby, I don't recall a trip to a pediatrician or any other doctor for the rest of the summer.

Our second-born arrived in the spring of my final year in medical school. This boy came into the world as if he had been shot out of a cannon. He wasn't unhappy with life, but he certainly made his roommates and the newborn nursery staff aware of his presence. I don't like to think that the head nurse of the nursery would inflict a vendetta upon this little troublemaker, but she discovered a rash she took as a sign that it was necessary to isolate our baby. So much for the pioneering work of the Grace New Haven Hospital in making the birthing experience as warm and delightful as possible by creating an atmosphere encouraging early bonding of mother and infant. Much later, I learned that this rash is called erythema toxicum, a transient condition likely due to exposure to some allergen in the amniotic fluid, and is not contagious.

Even though we were relatively inexperienced parents and certainly were not medical experts, it was soon apparent that this little guy was exceptionally alert and vigorous. This was confirmed with our first well visit to the pediatrician, who was a professor of pediatric hematology. He was not a stuffy scientist but a true physician we knew we could trust to level with us. I did notice a raised eyebrow as he attempted to overcome the intense muscle tone of our son as he assessed hip-joint health. In retrospect, he was probably concerned about a degree of spasticity (resembling cerebral palsy), but was wise enough to wait and see what a subsequent visit would reveal. This intense mental and physical activity persisted. He walked at nine months, and scared his parents and all my fellow residents in training by jumping down from great heights at age two. He was a high-hurdle champion in high school, did well academically, and became our anti-ADHD poster boy, because we recognized that genes aren't everything. It is what you do with what you've got, guided more by common sense than textbook learning, that really counts. (In *The Vitamin Cure for Children's Health Problems*,[1] we have an entire chapter on ADHD. I was in on the ground floor of this "man-made" diagnosis, and found no need for drugs. If you can find time, take a look at that chapter. Because the drug companies are pushing drugs on younger and younger children, parents of toddlers need to be armed with honest information. To quote from that book: "The genes we inherit determine the template for enzyme function—function that is influenced largely by vitamins, general nutrition, and environmental forces.")

I don't recall having overlooked any important health issues in my daughter during my remaining three years of medical school, possibly for failure to recognize them. I do wish my ideas of milk allergy had been better developed, but still I stumbled on my own onto good management for both of my children's severe allergies to cow's milk. I guess immunizations weren't a big deal, because I remember the name of our professor-pediatrician but little of what he did or what shots he inflicted. I don't think there were any given during the first year of life, and later just a diphtheria, whooping cough, and tetanus (DPT) vaccination or two. I cannot recall my daughter requiring any kind of urgent care.

As a young parent who hadn't completed medical school yet, the assumption might be made that I might not know enough to know when to go to the doctor. A big difference between then and now is that parents had a better understanding of both health and illness in those days. Basically, we new parents had been raised by parents who did not worry about taking their children to the doctor for minor health issues. They knew how to handle most common illnesses. I was prone to having colds that would "go down on my chest" (bronchitis). After applying a cloth soaked with camphorated oil to my chest and aiming a heat lamp at it for about twenty minutes, I can recall the "great expectorations" that followed. Or one could do the same with a doctor's office call, in which the doctor used a diathermy machine (that works similarly to microwave radiation) to break up the thick secretions. One doesn't see that sort of thing recommended too often any more, although Vicks Vaporub still contains camphor and is still advertised.

Of course, attitudes concerning health as well as health information often come from our parents and the whole "village" in which we are raised. Not all of that health information is good, even that derived from the doctors, then or now. My folks' bathroom medicine chest contained some "Dr. Porter's Antiseptic Healing Oil [oil, perhaps of the "snake" variety] Good for Man or Beast." It was carbolic acid (phenol), a foul-smelling substance with antiseptic qualities, to be rubbed on sore ligaments and other sore parts to provide pain relief and/or antisepsis. I would periodically get a real flare-up of my adenoid accompanying a respiratory infection. My folks would take me to a doctor who would put some of this magic solution on a finger of his gloved hand, make me promise not to bite and reach in with his index finger to press on the adenoid. He did this until either my gagging or biting caused him to cease fire. Strangely, it proved to be a fairly good treatment, perhaps because I was so relieved to have the treatment over with. I was sent to another doctor for allergy testing and a series of desensitizing shots for severe nasal allergy. The first time I ever wheezed was after one of these shots. When the doctor saw me struggling for breath, he ran down the hallway trying to get help from some other doctor who possibly might know what was going on—a real confidence buster, in my mind. I eventually got a shot of what I now must presume was adrenaline that brought me back to life. A few minutes later, the doctor allowed that I was fit enough to pedal the distance back home (over one mile). On the way, I formed my protest to my parents: enough already. At a younger age, another doctor put me on daily halibut liver oil capsules (with benefits similar to cod liver oil). So we had both the good and the not-so-good doctor care.

My point in all this background is that, in general, doctors were not considered to be godlike figures back then, even though some tried to convince parents that they were. My parents instilled a questioning attitude in me, similar to what they had. Some factors of good health came almost instinctively. Patients and doctors fed on the enlightenment they gained from each other. Both sides recognized the fact that neither knew it all. Growing up in that environment goes a long way toward developing discernment.

My naiveté as a new doctor, along with my personal experience, paid off, however, as I developed my concept of milk allergy. During my training at Los Angeles Children's Hospital I was given the privilege of conducting a sub-clinic for infants who had become allergic to a newly developed infant milk formula. The standard fare prior to this new formula was the evaporated milk formula, which had apparently subjected the milk proteins to enough heat to render them less allergenic. This sudden increase in the incidence of allergy caused many of the teachers of pediatrics to declare, "I'm getting allergic to milk allergy."

Along with the development of concepts of food allergy, nutrition concepts were rapidly changing at that time. A diet of whole-grain breads, sprouted seeds, beans, and grains, and other whole foods such as eggs, as well as an understanding of proper cooking of vegetables (minimal or zero) was encouraged and flourished, not only for its health benefits but also because it pleased the palate. I studied the health benefits of these tasty foods and realized that I had learned nearly none of this in medical school. There had been only two one-hour learning sessions covering two inconsequential subjects tangential to real nutrition. One discussed the benefit of feeding hogs peanuts, which made for a better fatty acid profile, which is good for the hog but does little for pork consumers. The other session covered an effect called entropy as it relates to the metabolism of food stuffs, which end up as carbon dioxide, water, and heat or energy. It was all expressed in a formula with a little "pyramid" at the beginning, signifying the mathematical symbol *delta*. In studying pathology, we skimmed over the vitamin-deficiency diseases—beriberi, scurvy, and rickets—and were taught the minimal doses of the appropriate vitamins necessary for life to continue. Additional nutrition courses (and the use of vitamins for disease prevention and reversal) were not offered or even considered.

Nowadays, the pharmaceutical industry attempts to pin diagnoses on ever-younger victims, and this needs to be said early in this book. From my long practice as a pediatrician, I think my story will be helpful to the reader: I have a lot of first-hand knowledge that I would like you to know about. We must get back the mutual respect between doctor and patient that comes from realizing that both are trying to do their best to work for healthy results. We are all individuals with individual needs, and cookie-cutter medicine will not offer the best solution for most of us. If we don't question procedures, we cannot hope to improve our children's health—we only reinforce what doesn't work.

I feel I waited far too long in today's medical environment before I began to question what I was being fed by a medical establishment that wished to keep things as they are—and still does. The fun of practice began with actually listening to my patients' parents, and I had even more fun listening to my older juvenile patients themselves. Out of the mouth of babes . . .

CHAPTER 2

IMMUNIZATIONS (MMR, INFLUENZA, PERTUSSIS, AND OTHERS)

Something has to put the brakes on the relentless push by vaccine manufacturers for approval of new vaccines by the U.S. Food and Drug Administration (FDA). Vaccines are neither foods nor drugs, yet this body accepts studies sponsored or run by the makers of vaccines that purportedly describe the safety and efficacy of their new product. Approval is almost rubber-stamped. Only data concerning the most severe reactions are collected or considered as important safety issues. It is necessary to study years of use to get a clear picture of efficacy, but very few controlled studies have been performed on the efficacy of individual vaccines.

When considering the current number of vaccinations now required for infants and children, let alone the number of vaccinations that are combined in one procedure, it is hard to believe how relatively few were required in the mid-fifties. Separately, each was developed earlier—the diphtheria vaccine in 1921; the pertussis (whooping cough) vaccine in 1930; and the tetanus toxoid vaccine, used extensively by the military during World War II. The three came together in the 1940s as the DPT vaccine. At the start of my pediatric practice in 1957, the DPT and the Salk inactivated ("killed") poliovirus vaccine, licensed just two years earlier, were the only two shots (a total of four antigens) that I—and my patients—had to deal with.

THE DPT VACCINE AND ITS RELATED DISEASES

I wasn't at all pleased with a fairly frequent side effect of the DPT: The development of a red, tender area at the injection site, high up in the buttocks. Crying told us that the area didn't just hurt from applied pressure but all the time. Fever accompanied the inflammation all too often. Parents asked, "Do we have to do more of these?" I reluctantly said, "Yes you do." The vaccine manufacturer either denied or minimized these complaints, so I thought it interesting when they changed the method of obtaining the proper pH (measurement of acidity). Of course the more of this vaccine I gave, the greater my chance was of encountering a "rare" side effect.

Two complications from the vaccinations may be rare, but they are terribly upsetting and scary for parents and (if honest) doctors alike. "Hypotonic-hyporesponsive" episodes were especially frightening. Immediately after the shot, the baby would become limp, pale, and almost lifeless—like it was struck down. When I witnessed this, I didn't time the interval until the baby came back to life, but it seemed an eternity. The second condition, called prolonged crying—for three hours or *more*—described only the objective part of the problem. The subjective part was the nature of the cry. I describe it as frantic, hysterical, and without purpose—an automatic response to brain irritation. Imagine the helpless feelings for a mother trying to comfort her little one, possibly when the *more* became *through most of the night*. There were, frequently, fever-related seizures, dismissed by the vaccine companies as occurring at an "acceptable" rate. As far as parents are concerned, having to witness just one febrile seizure is *un*acceptable. If an infant suffered either of these two serious effects of pertussis immunization, I would not administer any more of the series. This decision was completely supported by parents and gradually by the American Academy of Pediatrics (AAP).

In spite of strong evidence supporting the relationship of serious nervous system complications to the pertussis component of the vaccine, manufacturers, backed by authoritative bodies, consistently dismissed such claims. In 1994 the Institute of Medicine of the U.S. National Academy of Sciences stated, "If neurological symptoms occurred within seven days following vaccination, the evidence is compatible with the possibility of permanent brain damage in otherwise healthy children."[1] In spite of manufacturer denials of possible harm, the pertussis portion of the DPT was changed in 1991 to an acellular form, which they claimed would produce fewer side effects. (If it wasn't broke, why did they fix it?) DPT from then on became DTaP. It is now claimed that there is a marked reduction in the incidence of these side effects that used to be so rare that they were, supposedly, *of little importance*.

Pertussis (Whooping Cough)

Pertussis, or whooping cough, starts innocently with "cold" symptoms, progresses through a "dry" cough stage and moves on to the paroxysmal cough stage with the "whoop." The patient, in the characteristic "whoop" stage, has paroxysms of coughing in which the cough is so hard and continuous that the patient becomes completely out of air, then desperately draws in a breath accompanied by a loud "whoop" made noticeable from inflammation of the larynx. This often is followed with vomiting which, reflexively, helps a little in clearing the respiratory tree. When the whooping stage subsides, a reversion to the disturbing and persistent "dry" cough takes place, making the total illness last as long as six to ten weeks. In an epidemic, atypical signs in any age group can occur, such as not having a "whoop" phase, making diagnosis more ambiguous. Certain strains of adenovirus can also produce a nasty paroxysmal cough that hangs on, further confusing the issue. Confirmatory laboratory tests are cumbersome and often fraught with false negative results; so are usually skipped. The organism is sensitive to the antibiotic erythromycin or its up-to-date derivatives, which can be used for prevention. Once a patient is in the "paroxysmal cough" stage, however, the antibiotic is unable to get to the bacteria trapped in secretions of the respiratory tree and can provide little improvement.

An argument for pertussis vaccination is based on the seriousness of the disease. Infants, vaccinated or not, who contract pertussis can eventually be found in critical condition. The incidence of pneumonia in infants with pertussis was reported as high as 20 percent over a period from 1990 to 1999, according to State Health reports published in the 2003 Red Book of the Committee on Infectious Diseases of the AAP.[2] A rare but very worrisome result of the disease is obvious brain involvement with encephalopathy or seizures. In those early days, I administered pooled gamma globulin by injection to an infected infant, hoping that it contained a high level of antibodies to the pertussis organism. Gamma globulin is no longer available and would probably be ineffective if it were. See below for finding that the antibody response to the newer vaccine is poor.

After being in the shot business long enough, I observed that the disease could be bad, but that pertussis vaccination was not the preventive measure it was purported to be. Many appropriately vaccinated children still would succumb to clinical pertussis during an epidemic. It is nearly impossible to get reliable figures of efficacy of the pertussis vaccine in our country due to inadequate documentation of illness and/or immunization records. But in the United Kingdom, which has national record keeping and reporting, there were over 200,000 cases of pertussis in fully vaccinated individuals during the period of 1970–1990. This figure comes from the U.K. Community Disease Surveillance Centre, their equivalent of our Centers for Disease Control and Prevention (CDC).

As I am writing, there are extensive outbreaks of pertussis in the United States; Montana, like New York and California, is having outbreaks of pertussis here and there, causing health officials to encourage both young and old to get their pertussis vaccination. Health officials are of one mind: immunize everybody—and they claim an 85 percent efficiency for the vaccine. I don't know how they could possibly arrive at that optimistic figure. One official talked about "medication." There is no medication. Perhaps she was referring to antibiotic prophylaxis to prevent spread of pertussis to an infant in the household. Such a fear smear included a report of one death of a baby in Idaho. This has folks clamoring for the poorly effective vaccination. The Missoula, Montana Health Official believes that the new acellular vaccine is not as effective as the old version, and is the only official attempt to obtain immunization histories. In Seattle's large epidemic, over half the victims were "fully immunized." Yet hysteria wins every time.

Our neighbor, Washington State, is among several states experiencing a pertussis epidemic. All public health officials are in agreement and are pushing vaccination booster shots for middle school students, high school students, and even for adults. The acellular DTaP pertussis vaccine, designed for adults, was licensed for use in infants and children in 2003. Many people's knowledge of the DPT vaccination is woefully out of date, because the old DPT gave good protection but had more (and sometimes) terrible side effects. To my knowledge there have been no studies of efficacy regarding the new version of the vaccine, nor has there been full disclosure about its side effects.

As this is being written, more candid reporting concerning pertussis vaccine is appearing but this sort of information has to be searched for, since it is never part of the media treatment of pertussis. The following are examples:

Dr. Paul Offit of Vaccination Education Department of Philadelphia Children's Hospital describes the early DPT in wide use in the 1940s, which contained the pertussis organism treated with formaldehyde, creating inactivated pertussis toxins (toxoids), as highly effective but fraught with serious side effects caused by some 3,000 abnormal bacterial proteins it contained. By eliminating these proteins, the acellular vaccine employed in 1997 reduced the serious side effects but also proved to be not nearly as effective. My take on this is that the standard medical solution seems to favor the reduction of side effects over the question of effectiveness and to propose *giving more shots in the hope that "more" is better.* Some experts support the idea that side effects have been reduced; some do not.

Dr. James Cherry discussed California's 2010 pertussis epidemic in an article in *Pediatrics,* the official journal of the American Academy of Pediatrics.[3] "Some preadolescents' booster strength may have waned because of replacement of *whole pertussis vaccine* with the *less efficacious acellular vaccine,*" he wrote. "Most vulnerable were babies too young for vaccination." (Makes me wonder about the immune status of a young mother who "grew up" with the acellular vaccine.

With the old vaccine, maternal antibodies protected newborns and young infants. Certainly they were not so vulnerable.) In the one-to-eighteen-year age group, 9 percent were not immunized. Does this mean that 91 percent were? This is the first admission I have run across that questions whether we might be insisting that everyone, including adults, get a subpar vaccine. Since an infant infected with pertussis might not whoop or a child might not ever develop a whoop but just remain in the catarrhal (runny nose) phase for weeks, pertussis cases are largely unreported. An infant who does not whoop can still need hospitalization in order to properly manage life-threatening tenacious secretions.

YOUR CHILD'S AMAZING BODY

- In just one day, a baby cries an average of 133 minutes.
- In just one square inch of his skin, there are seventy-seven feet (not a misprint!) of nerves and nineteen feet of blood vessels.
- When she is a grown adult, her bones will still be 50 percent water.

In your child's lifetime:
- His eyes will blink 450 million times.
- She will breathe 650 million times.
- He will grow 1,000 layers of skin.
- Her nails will have grown seven feet.
- He will lose seventy miles of hair from his head.
- Her heart will beat 2,500,000,000 times! (In one minute, a hamster's heart beats about 500 times, and a whale's about 9 times.)

By age seventy:
- He will have shed 105 pounds of skin cells.
- And, very likely, will be a grandparent, like us.

No Real Choice?

The justified fear that health officers have is that infants too young to be immunized might be exposed to pertussis. We used to be able to treat an infant with pertussis with administration of intramuscular (IM) pooled gamma globulin, which had a high level of pertussis anti- bodies, but this treatment is no longer available. And, as mentioned above, antibiotic treatment doesn't work once the patient is in the whooping stage because the blood-borne antibiotic can't get through to the infected and secretion-filled bronchi and trachea. The current *treatment* for infants is antibiotic *prophylaxis* to prevent exposure. Prevention being the best treatment has encouraged health authorities to recommend prophylactic antibiotics to household members when there is a vulnerable infant in the house. So in a pertussis outbreak health authorities are left only with antibiotic prophylaxis, hygienic measures to prevent spread of disease, and vaccinating everybody, even adults, with a vaccine that many of us think is pretty poor and has not been carefully studied. Depiction of an infant with pertussis is a pow- erful incentive for the vaccination program, and I don't see how we can counter this until some honest studies are brought to light. If immu- nization histories are obtained, as was done in Seattle recently and showed that over 50 percent of victims were "fully immunized," it should certainly encourage a hard look at the current vaccine. But change is slow. Yes, consider every alternative, but I am afraid that we are trapped in the protocol of the experts, who can even shut down school attendance and keep unimmunized kids out of school.

And it all changes fast. I (RKC) have two "immunization" folders. In one version I have thirty-five antigens in sixteen to twenty-three separate shots, which are inflicted before or at the time of the child's first birthday. In another (2011) version, I have thirty-seven antigens in sixteen to twenty-one shots. The variability in the number of shots depends on the variety of combinations of antigens that are possible. It all changes every year as governmental and medical authorities convince themselves that more antigens can be given at earlier ages, that repeated doses are needed more frequently than previously thought, and that more combinations are acceptable. Let's just say it is a mess, way overdone, and "I'm mad as hell and I'm not going to take it anymore."

One morning the headline was "200 Cases of Pertussis Statewide." When I was Health Officer in our county, I'll bet we had 200 cases during an epidemic in our county alone. Most were mild cases and parents didn't run their kids to the doctor, especially after being told that there was no active treatment and that accurate confirmation could only be made through a nasal-pharyngeal swab passed through a youngster's nose. At present, officials downplay the incidence of "mild" cases and only report confirmed (by an easier test) cases—no matter the intensity of clinical signs. This idea was strengthened by a previous citation about the California epidemic.[4] Folks simply are not going to run to the doctor if not sick, especially if there is no insurance coverage. On the other hand, an infant can have serious difficulty from the tenacious secretions in the respiratory tree. Don't self-diagnose. Rather, get professional evaluation. It is hard to make progress with the pertussis dilemma without more honest evaluation.

And here it is: The old DPT gave good protection but had more, and sometimes terrible, side effects. So, acellular DTaP pertussis vaccine, designed for adults, was licensed for use in infants and children in 2003. It is generally regarded as safer. To my knowledge there have been no studies of efficacy—by all appearances, it is less effective—nor has there been openness about side effects (the piece below may be the first—a hopeful beginning).

PERTUSSIS VACCINE MAY BE INADEQUATE

Pertussis vaccine is effective about half of the time for all children, and only 24 percent of the time for kids ages eight to twelve. The authors of one study wrote that, "despite widespread childhood vaccination against Bordetella pertussis, disease remains prevalent. It has been suggested that acellular vaccine may be less effective than previously believed. During a large outbreak, we examined the incidence of pertussis and effectiveness of vaccination in a well-vaccinated, well-defined community. We identified 171 cases of clinical pertussis, 132 of which were in pediatric patients. (Of these, 81 percent were up-to-date on recommended whooping cough shots.) The vaccine effectiveness was 41 percent, 24 percent, and 79 percent for children aged two to seven years, eight to twelve years, and thirteen to eighteen years, respectively."[1]

In an interview, Dr. David Witt, one of the study authors, said, "We have a real belief that the durability (of the vaccine) is not what was imagined. . . What was very surprising was the majority of cases were in fully vaccinated children."[2]

References

1. Witt, M. A., P. H. Katz, D. J. Witt. "Unexpectedly Limited Durability of Immunity Following Acellular Pertussis Vaccination in Preadolescents in a North American Outbreak." *Clin Infect Dis* 54(12) (Jun 2012):1730–1735.

2. Grens, K. "Whooping Cough Vaccine Fades in Pre-Teens: Study." Reuters, Apr 3, 2012. http://www.reuters.com/article/2012/04/03/us-whoopingcough-idUSBRE8320 TM20120403 (accessed Oct 2012).

Diphtheria

I (RKC), like most physicians of my era, had never seen a case of diphtheria, but we certainly knew that it had been a terrible scourge in earlier days—snatching the lives of infants and children. We attributed, without question, success in *eliminating* this dreaded disease to vaccination. Then what happened? People in the early, subclinical period of the disease who traveled to our shores from endemic areas across the seas presented the disease to susceptible U.S. citizens and created quite a problem. Of course, with aircraft travel, we will find this phenomenon occurring more frequently in our ever-smaller world, since there will always be a body of susceptible people even in a well immunized population.

POLIO

Aside from the diphtheria vaccine, the Salk polio vaccine (inactivated, or killed, polio virus given by injection) was the only other vaccine I used

VITAMIN C AS PREVENTION AND TREATMENT OF PERTUSSIS

Bordetella pertussis is the whooping cough bacteria. Vitamin C is, at saturation doses, an effective antibiotic. Vitamin C given by intravenous (IV) infusion is the fastest acting and most effective method of administration. Intramuscular (IM) injections are next quickest. Aggressive (very frequent) oral C therapy is the most inexpensive third option for home care. But it must be emphasized that the preferred method is IV or IM, either or both of which may be demanded by the patient, parent, or guardian. "Demand" is certainly the right word.

Making a demand does not guarantee getting it—not by a long shot. (Ha!) If IV/IM administration is not available, vitamin C can be given orally to good effect. However, it must be given *very* frequently, literally every ten to fifteen minutes that the patient is awake in sufficient quantity to produce "bowel tolerance" (near-diarrhea). The quantity given orally may need to exceed 1,200 milligrams (mg) vitamin C per kilogram of body weight per day. That is over 600 mg of vitamin C per pound of baby. Small amounts will not produce results.

Questions parents usually ask are: Why so much? How can you get that much down a little child? Is it safe?

The answers, in order, are:

1. Saturation of vitamin C has therapeutic effect; low doses do not. We discuss dosage later, in Chapter 14, High-Dose Vitamin C Therapy.

2. Use sweet juice (or any sweet liquid, really) to hide the taste of the dissolved vitamin C powder. Vitamin C powder (crystals) is readily available in health food stores and on the Internet.

3. Compared to literally any medical treatment, yes, it is safe.

This approach is indeed work for the parent, but rearing children, especially when they are sick, is already a huge amount of work. The work is worth it when you can have a healthier child sooner. One needs to also bear in mind that when choosing care, the standard is not perfection; the standard is the alternative. Antibiotics, cough medicines, and medical therapy in general have nearly insignificant effect in pertussis treatment and no specific allopathic (traditional Western medicine) treatment is known.

Vitamin C has been successfully used to treat whooping cough since 1936, when doctors reported that "In 66 [of 81] cases [we saw] . . . reduction of lip cyanosis in coughing attacks; . . . [disappearance of] attacks with breathing difficulty, vomiting and recurrence; . . . also the number of cough attacks diminished. Patients became lively, had good appetite and the convalescence progressed very satisfactorily. Of special mention were 3 serious cases of pertussis pneumonia . . . which were deemed as having lethal outcome. Through our therapy, the children were clearly improved after 2–3 weeks and finally healed." The therapy was injected vitamin C.[1]

In 1937, another team of physicians wrote "Ascorbic acid definitely shortens the paroxysmal stage of the disease, particularly if relatively large doses are used early in the disease."[2] This observation was followed with this even more striking observation: "Saturation of whooping cough patients with ascorbic acid decreases markedly the intensity, number and duration of the characteristic symptoms."[3]

In 1938, another team of doctors wrote that in a "series of twenty-six cases of whooping cough, cevitamic acid [ascorbic acid] seemed to be strikingly effective in relieving and checking the symptoms in all but two of the cases . . . . It is our opinion that it should be given further trial in all cases of whooping cough regardless of the age of the patient, or the length of time already elapsed since the original symptoms."[4]

All this before WW II began. Imagine that.

More recently, Frederick R. Klenner, M.D., has provided much information about the use of large doses of vitamin C in preventing and treating many diseases. His papers are easily obtainable through an Internet search. Dr. Klenner asserted that "ascorbic acid (vitamin C) is the safest and most valuable substance available to the physician." He also said that patients should be given large doses of vitamin C "in all pathological conditions while the physician ponders the diagnosis."[5]

"I have used Dr. Klenner's methods on hundreds of patients," said pediatrician Lendon H. Smith, M.D. "He is right."[6]

May we say again that more details will be found later in this book in Chapter 14. Additional books and articles by Frederick Klenner that may be of interest can be found in the special section "A Brief Listing of Titles by Frederick R. Klenner" in the Recommended Reading at the end of this book.

References

1. Otani, T. "Concerning the Vitamin C Therapy of Whooping-Cough." Klinische Wochenschrift, 15(51) (Dec 1936):1884–1885. Available online at http://www.whale.to/a/otani1936.html (accessed April 2013).

2. Ormerod, M. J., B. M. Unkauf. "Ascorbic Acid (Vitamin C) Treatment of Whooping Cough." *Can Med Assoc J* 37(2) (Aug 1937):134–136. Available online at http://www.ncbi.nlm.nih.gov/pmc/articles/PMC1562195/pdf/canmedaj00527-0084.pdf (accessed April 2013).

3. Ormerod, M. J., B. M. Unkauf, F. D. White. "A Further Report on the Ascorbic Acid Treatment of Whooping Cough." *Can Med Assoc J* 37(3) (Sep 1937):268–272. Available online at http://www.ncbi.nlm.nih.gov/pmc/articles/PMC536087/pdf/canmedaj00183-0060.pdf (accessed April 2013).

4. Vermillion, E. L., G. E. Stafford. "A Preliminary Report on the Use of Cevitamic Acid in the Treatment of Whooping Cough." *J Kansas Med Soc* 34(11) (Nov 1938):469, 479.

5. Saul, A. W. "Hidden in Plain Sight: The Pioneering Work of Frederick Robert Klenner, M.D." *J Orthomolecular Med* 22(1) (2007):31–38. Available online at http://orthomolecular.org/library/jom/2007/pdf/2007-v22n01-p031.pdf and http://www.doctoryourself.com/klennerbio.html (accessed Oct 2012).

6. Ibid.

early on. I was pleased with reports of its effectiveness, and I had not encountered any drawbacks to its use. Poliomyelitis, or infantile paralysis, is a horrible disease. Fear of it was substantial and deserved. Pictures of children in braces or of President Roosevelt in a wheelchair brought out many emotions in onlookers, especially the fear of not knowing who would be the next victim or what we could do to not become (or have our children become) that victim. Showing a person in an "iron lung" was the epitome of fear production. With bulbar polio, nerve signals to the diaphragm were disrupted. The patient was placed in this steel cylinder with a tight seal around the neck, allowing his head to protrude. Since the patient's diaphragm was paralyzed and could not develop negative pressure to allow incoming air to fill the lungs, the machine had to take over this function. No one with even a twinge of feeling for his fellow man could allow this to continue. Try to imagine the vicissitudes of this victim. Ordinary functions of living, such as eating and elimination, were no longer ordinary. It was truly remarkable that this vaccine was developed so rapidly and was proving effective.

Epidemics in the U.S. peaked in the summer and early fall and seemed to be selective for physically active adults and children. Transmission through flies was suspected, which at least led investigators to the fecal-oral method of transmission. Later studies found that infection is very widespread during a siege, with a large majority of patients showing either influenza-like symptoms or none at all, and only 1 percent showing that the virus entered the nervous system. The virus enters the gastrointestinal system through contaminated food or drink, then goes to the lymphoid tissue of that system (such as the tonsils) and on into the bloodstream, where it can reside for weeks. Even though it rarely gets into the nervous system from there, it can produce aseptic meningitis (affecting the covering of the brain) with symptoms of stiff neck and headache. Thankfully, this is often short lived and has no other nervous system involvement. When the virus *does* get into the nervous system, paralytic polio begins with these symptoms and many more, including fever, weakness, muscle pain, and loss of reflexes. The virus destroys motor nerves (those related to producing motion), most often in the spinal cord but in rare cases in the cranial nerves (bulbar polio). These nerves can not recover. "Treatment" is designed to allow

HOMEOPATHY AND PERTUSSIS

If you suspect that parts of this book will be unusual, here is your first confirmation from me (AWS):

Samuel Hahnemann, M.D., the founder of homeopathic medicine, successfully treated pertussis with one single dose of Drosera rotundifulia in the thirtieth centessimal (30C) potency.[1] Hahnemann specifically wrote in his *Material Medica Pura* (Volume 6, 1827) that "a single such dose is quite sufficient for the homoeopathic cure if epidemic whooping-cough."

It is possible but not especially easy to set aside a report like that, especially considering the source. Christian Friedrich Samuel Hahnemann was a fully and conventionally qualified physician, earning his M.D. with honors in 1779. He also mastered at least nine languages and became widely known as an expert medical translator.

Homeopaths generally suggest that one does not administer a homeopathic remedy concurrently with other medicine or its effectiveness will be reduced. Virtually no harm to the patient would occur even if casually administered. This is an attractive aspect of homeopathy.

The problem is that there is little if any conventional scientific explanation as to how this treatment could possibly work. First of all, Drosera rotundifolia is the sundew plant. The name is derived from the Greek *droseros* meaning "dewy, watery" and the Latin *rotundus,* "round," and *folius,* meaning "leaf." Furthermore, a 30C homeopathic potency means that the substance has been diluted one part in one hundred . . . thirty successive times. That would probably only leave a few molecules of the plant in the remedy. It is easy (and routine) to dismiss homeopathy at this point, and modern medicine has done exactly that.

Still, there remains a poser. If the remedy is so dilute as to be useless, how can it harm? An absence of danger removes the biggest reason to not try it. I know a family that did use Drosera for a child's whooping cough. It worked exactly as Hahnemann said it would, 150 years after he said it. This is at the very least intriguing.

Homeopathic remedies are government regulated, but usually do not require a prescription because of well over a century of established safety. ". . . Homeopathic drugs are subject to the Food, Drug, and Cosmetic Act and regulations issued by FDA . . . [as] published in the Homeopathic Pharmacopoeia of the United States (HPUS). The criteria for inclusion in the HPUS require that a homeopathic drug product be determined by HPCUS to be safe and effective and to be prepared according to the specifications of the HPUS general pharmacy section."[2]

The chief homeopathic side effect is a slight aggravation of symptoms immediately before relief. Such "provings" are possible with repeated doses, but are not likely. According to data collected by the American Association of Poison Control Centers (AAPCC), there are zero deaths per year from conventional homeopathic remedies.[3]

More information about homeopathy will be found with an Internet search and by reading practical, informative books such as John H. Clarke's *The Prescriber* and Harris L. Coulter's *Homeopathic Science and Modern Medicine.*

Important caution: Common sense dictates the need for genuine care in dealing with whooping cough or any serious illness. Consult a physician before proceeding with these, or any other self-care approaches.

References

1. Boericke, W. *Materia Medica with Repertory,* 9th Edition, Boericke & Tafel, 1927. 258–259.

2. Borneman, J. P., R. I. Field. "Regulation of Homeopathic Drug Products." *Am J Health-Syst Pharm* 63(1) (Jan 1, 2006):86–91. Available online at http://www.hylands.com/news/regulation.php (accessed Oct 2012).

3. American Association of Poison Control Centers. Poison Data. Annual Reports. http://www.aapcc.org/annual-reports/ (accessed Oct 2012).

adjacent muscle groups to partially compensate for the loss. Thus, braces were sometimes employed for lower-limb paralysis.

The Sabin oral polio vaccine containing all three strains of poliovirus has been in play since 1963. It seemed to be doing a good job until it was discovered that the live virus could revert to a paralytic form in geographic areas with low vaccination coverage. This led to a return to the injectable Salk vaccine (IVP), which could also be combined with other injectable vaccines. Either form produces excellent immunity in different ways. The IVP does a better job of preventing the poliovirus from entering the nervous system. The oral version does a better job of providing intestinal immunity. The oral vaccine is more suitable in polio-endemic areas of the world that have less stringent hygiene. In our world, where there are pockets of unimmunized people and danger of the oral live vaccine creating paralytic illness, the IVP is best.

IVP seems to provide very long-term immunity, contributing to claims from the CDC that polio was eliminated in the U.S. in 1994. Since we are in good shape in respect to polio infection, I see no reason for starting immunization at such an early age (the recommended schedule of two months, four months and six months). Spare the immature immune system from working overtime.

OTHER "CHILDHOOD" DISEASES AND THEIR VACCINATIONS

The young child's immune system is further pressed by many additional vaccinations, some of which we think are of questionable value. Even immunizations that have merit are given too soon. Why so young? The theory is that infants need all the shots they can get, right away, to keep from getting all those illnesses. Our view is that the infant's own immune system is weakened by too many shots too early.

Measles

With only the drawbacks to pertussis vaccination, I got along reasonably well with the concept of vaccinating my patients until the first measles vaccine was approved in 1963. Here we have a case of meaning well but getting a poor result. President John F. Kennedy's older sister, Rose, apparently was somewhat retarded and had some related behavior problems. When she was twenty, her father was swayed by the new science of lobotomy (literally surgically cutting through the connecting nerve fibers of the brain's two hemispheres) and allowed his daughter to undergo this procedure. In short, it made her worse, and she was institutionalized. The family loved Rose and was terribly affected by this tragedy. Knowing that measles could lead to brain damage, even though rarely, President Kennedy listened carefully when his medical advisors apprised him of the possibilities of a measles vaccine. Research and development was hurried along, and the vaccine got into the hands of U.S. doctors with the president's blessing. Prior to that time, gamma globulin had been used for passive immunity (the blood of people who had had measles contained high levels of measles antibodies in their gamma globulin, which could be extracted from donated blood) when exposure was fresh and before real measles signs had begun. This could give temporary protection and diminish the severity of a measles infection. With the development of this new vaccine, doctors were instructed to give, in shot form, the new killed-virus vaccine in one arm and gamma globulin in the other.

Since the antibodies to measles in the gamma globulin could block stimulation of antibody formation from the killed vaccine, many physicians refused to give this combination. We were thankful later that we had made the right choice for our patients when reports in following years told of cases of "atypical measles" in those who had received this vaccine. They suffered serious measles pneumonia, pleural effusion (not responsive to antibiotic treatment), and swelling of the extremities.

Until the measles vaccination was developed, most people had the natural disease before reaching adulthood and had developed lifetime immunity as a result. This is also the case with a chicken pox or rubella (German measles) infection. Vaccination disease prevention is much weaker than that derived from natural infection. Vaccinated individuals, when immune protection is fading, are prone to develop disease that is much more severe than that naturally acquired in childhood. In parts of the third world where vitamin A deficiency is prevalent, blindness caused by measles and severe pneumonia rank high. This can be modified by providing massive doses of vitamin A, which greatly reduces the incidence of these complications.

Which brings us to the next vaccine problem. Chicken pox in a pregnant woman can lead to deformities in her fetus, as can a rubella infection. Little attention was given to rubella in the pre-vaccination era. You caught it as a child, got to miss a few days of school, and life went on. Congenital rubella is hard to relate to such a mild childhood infectious disease. It is horrible. Infection transmitted to the developing fetus can affect development of the eyes, the heart, neurological system components, and the blood-forming system. This translates to cataracts or blindness, all sorts of congenital heart lesions, hearing loss, or mental retardation. The earlier in the pregnancy (even before pregnancy is suspected) that congenital infection occurs, the worse the outcome. The numbers of cases per thousand might not be high, but something that can so drastically alter a developing life must be dealt with.

Knowing that childhood infection was a good thing in the case of rubella, pediatricians encouraged "rubella parties." Since girls are more social than boys, it was relatively easy to get a group of girls not fortunate enough to have had rubella yet over to the house of a girl enjoying the peak of the disease. I had a girl in my practice who had unsuccessfully attended many such parties and was approaching womanhood, so I gave her the rubella vaccine that was licensed in 1967. Later, she developed what was a dead ringer for "rheumatoid monarticular arthritis" (arthritis in a single joint) in one hip joint and later "uveitis" (inflammation in the eye), which is typically associated with this type of arthritis—all later attributed to that first rubella vaccine.

Live virus versions were developed for both measles and rubella. A measles rubella (MR) vaccine (both live virus components) was used in practice after 1967 and before the 1971 measles, mumps, and rubella (MMR) vaccine was marketed. At first it was given at eighteen months of age, then at fifteen months, and later there was a push to give it between one year and fifteen months. Immunity developed by the vaccine was expected to last a lifetime. After a resurgence of measles in the U.S. in 1988, studies revealed that in many people immunity waned to insufficient levels in as short a time as eight years. As a result a booster shot for measles, using the 1971 MMR, was recommended (and in many instances demanded) for junior-high-aged children.

Mumps

The "M" added to MR means "mumps." Different killed vaccines for mumps were in effect from 1950 to 1978. None produced lasting immunity and were sparingly used for the reasons described below.

Mumps isn't too debilitating, but it can distort the face with swelling of the parotid glands (below the ear and under the jaw). It can be quite uncomfortable, but fortunately it is not long lasting. Rarely, it can infect other than salivary glands. It often can be detected in cerebrospinal fluid, but few have symptoms of nervous system infection. When it infects a testicle, discomfort and swelling are considerable. From a look at this condition, one would expect dire consequences. Fortunately, resulting sterility is rare.[5] Nevertheless, we don't sit idle when one's manhood is at stake. Proactive action for any child having reached adolescence without having had mumps is an excuse for giving mumps protection. Unfortunately, we no longer are allowed to wait but dive right in with an MMR shot for all youngsters twelve to fifteen months of age. At least the vaccine was upgraded to a "live" virus type.

With the MR replaced by the MMR, it is difficult to drop the unnecessary (in my mind) mumps component from immunization schedule of those so young. I urge working toward this goal. I can see no harm in getting the MR back to the old eighteen month regimen. However, with the present vaccines having been in place for such a long time, it is hard to predict how much this upset of natural immunity could result in disease in a poorly vaccinated area.

Hib

In 1985 the vaccine industry took off. A bacterium, *Haemophilus influenzae*, mostly the B strains (Hib), caused both common and serious disease in infants and toddlers: middle ear infections, croup, epiglottitis, and meningitis. Croup due to this bacterial infection was severe. Worse was epiglottitis. The epiglottis is a flap that, in the act of swallowing, closes off the larynx to prevent substances in the throat from getting into the wrong "tube." If the epiglottis becomes infected it swells and rapidly blocks the airway—a medical emergency. The Hib organism was the leading cause of bacterial meningitis in infants and toddlers. It was one of the three most prominent bacterial causes of middle ear infections, which on rare occasions can progress to meningitis. Many young children "carried" this organism in their nose and throat without becoming ill. They were effective spreaders of disease in settings like a preschool. The need for a vaccine was great; especially since more little germ spreaders than ever were getting together in day-care centers and exchanging germs.

The Hib vaccine was on the market and recommended by all the authoritative bodies to be given not before age two. Pediatricians scratched their collective heads and asked, "How then are infants going to gain benefit from this vaccine?" It was later determined that a good immune response to this type of vaccine didn't take place until after eighteen months. This revelation came late; in 1988 the vaccine was discontinued. Within the next two years a new vaccine that stimulated the formation of antibodies to a different portion of the bacterium was created, and was put to use in 1990. It is claimed that the carrier rate has declined markedly, as have the rates for the serious diseases associated with Hib. Unless I could be shown that there was an unacceptable rate of serious disease in infants (up to one year of age) in the pre-vaccination era, I would like to see the vaccination schedule changed from starting at two months to starting between six months to one year at the earliest.

TO VACCINATE OR NOT TO VACCINATE

She is fine, but my (AWS) granddaughter experienced a fairly severe vaccination reaction just days ago as of my writing this. The good news is that her parents prepared for the event. She has taken vitamin C supplements every day since birth, and more C before and after vaccination appointments. My daughter brought her baby's 103.5° fever down 2 degrees with vitamin C alone in just a couple of hours, and 4 degrees total in eight hours. This was not a chance effect, as the fever fluctuated inversely with the vitamin C intake. Every time the C "wore off" (about two hours), the fever climbed and the child was fretful and not herself. Then Mom gave her more C and down came the fever again, and she was fine. Dr. Archie Kalokerinos was right. (We will discuss his work in the sudden infant death syndrome [SIDS] chapter.)

I raised my own children without vaccination. This was neither

a light decision nor an easy path. When I registered my unvaccinated children for public school, the school nurse confirmed that
my religious exemption was acceptable. I was further informed that,
should there be an epidemic at the school, my children would have
to stay home.

Wait a minute: If the other kids are vaccinated, what do they have
to worry about? And if there *is* a worry, maybe those vaccinations
aren't all they are cracked up to be. If their shots are so great, then
why send my kids home? I would like to think that the school medical staff was actually saying that to protect my children from any
outbreak. But that doesn't fit either, as contagious diseases are generally contagious before symptoms erupt.

How come the unvaccinated are not all sick all the time? Consider
the Amish. They should, by the standards of school-district doctoring,
all be dead, or paralyzed with polio, or crippled with lockjaw
(tetanus), or at least plagued by a never-ending bevy of rampant life-
threatening epidemics. Well, they aren't. If they were, you can be
sure that our pharmaphilic (drug-lovin') news media would be quick
to report that entire populations of "religious extremists" have been
wiped out by their rejection of modern medicine.

That has not happened. And it's not because the Amish are isolated from the "germs" of others, either. The Amish maintain frequent contact with the rest of society. My parents lived right in the
Amish epicenter: Lancaster, Pennsylvania. Everywhere they went,
unvaccinated Amish people were there, too: horses, black buggies,
and all. The Amish are not an isolated community and they are not a
vaccinated community, yet they generally are a healthy community.
Ever see a bunch of sickly farmers work horses in the field or raise a
barn? No way. And they'd be an even healthier lifestyle model if
they'd stop raising tobacco.

The practical answer for society in general? Natural immunity
through optimum diet, and stand-by heavy-hitter therapy with
huge doses of vitamin C. To think the needle alone is going to protect your children is a silly as thinking that drugs will magically make
you healthy.

THE FLOOD GATES OPEN

In 1991 new vaccines appeared in a rapid-fire manner, starting with the hepatitis B vaccination: in 1995, a varicella (chicken pox) vaccine, and a hepatitis A vaccine. In 1998 a rotavirus vaccine was introduced, withdrawn the next year, and reintroduced with a better version in 2006. This was a frenetic period. It is hard to overlook the thinking, or lack of it, that prompted the development and introduction into recommendations for these vaccines.

Hepatitis B is transmitted through blood or "body fluids" (polite term for mainly semen and cervical secretions). In practical terms, the risk is high in a culture of promiscuous sex and/or "shooting up" with contaminated needles. Many, who are chronically infected, develop liver cancer. At the time the vaccine was introduced, the only plausible reason in the pediatric literature to give the vaccine to a child was that many chronically infected Vietnamese and Cambodian immigrants were living in extremely crowded conditions (to save rent money), making transmission more likely. Extrapolated from this was the recommendation for a series of three shots, starting with the newborn— *all* newborns. I doubt very much that there have been many conversations between a doctor and a new mother about the possibility of postponing these shots until they see how the child-rearing thing is going. There is always the hope that the child will not choose dangerous behavior as a lifestyle. I feel strongly that this vaccination should not even be considered before the teen years, and then only with parental consent.

In pre-vaccination days, chicken pox (varicella) was an expected childhood disease of little consequence. Most children of elementary-school age had been infected before junior-high age. Since the virus is easily spread, most susceptible children got the disease each spring. I don't recall seeing infants with chicken pox in our county, an indication that the mother retained strong immunity from her own childhood infection and passed it on to her fetus. Complications were rare but serious. Out of thousands of reported cases, I had only one case that developed cerebellar ataxia (a transient balance problem) in the pre-vaccination era. This unusual complication was alarming, but fortunately it quickly resolved. Shingles (herpes zoster infection resurgence) can appear when immunity wanes or the immune system is not up to snuff, usually in older folks, but occasionally in children. It is interesting that two such diverse disorders are due to the same virus. The chicken pox virus mostly leaves the scene after a bout of chicken pox, but some hides out in nerve cells. Just what activates the virus to move down the nerve axon to create a painful, burning skin rash along the distribution of the nerve is poorly understood. The nerves running along the underside of the ribs are a common site. Children don't seem to suffer much if they do get shingles, but adults can suffer from intense pain for months after the skin lesions have dried (within five to seven days). (The other herpes, *herpes simplex*, behaves similarly, as it causes a periodic outbreak of a "cold sore.")

Authorities are concerned that "as more and more children are immunized and wild-type varicella (caught from other people) decreases, a higher proportion of varicella cases will occur in immunized people as a "breakthrough disease."[6] They believe that this could be due to vaccine failure. But this can happen with any program that does not immunize everyone unless, perhaps, the vaccine is so effective that there is lifelong immunity (like that claimed for the polio vaccination). I wish this vaccine had never been developed, but we can't go back. We have to adjust to the fact that the population is only partially immunized—and we have no idea of the length of protection.

HERD IMMUNITY

"Herd immunity" is a concept that many immunologists adhere to. It is believed that a population will be well protected from a "childhood infection" disease if 85 percent of "susceptibles" are immunized. The theory can never be proven, because *vaccinated* individuals are not necessarily immunized, due to unique differences in immune response. I doubt if there will ever be a controlled study. This would require baseline tests for antibody levels, done before an epidemic strikes, to determine who is truly immunized. More attention needs to be given to how we can strengthen our immune systems. Proper nutrition with vitamin supplementation provides the best known boost.

We now jump to 1998 and the introduction of the rotavirus vaccine mentioned above. Rotavirus is the foremost cause of the vomiting-diarrhea illnesses of infants and young children. It, like a host of other viruses that affect the gut, is spread hand to mouth (fecal-oral). The bad news is that it is capable of causing severe diarrhea in infants, who can readily become dehydrated. The good news is that, if an infant can get through that first infection easily, immunity is developed that gets stronger with each subsequent infection. This illness is so widespread that nearly all three-year-olds have developed strong immunity. Adults can be infected but rarely have symptoms. (Adult are more apt to gain misery from a Norwalk virus. Add this infection, acquired on a cruise, to seasickness, and one is truly sick.) I have always hated it when one of these vomiting-diarrhea bugs would hit town (yes, there are others). If a suitable regimen of fluid maintenance is started early, no problem. But it does have to start *early* with an infant.

Well, the new oral vaccine didn't work. It sometimes promoted a very serious side effect of intussusception, in which a segment of bowel has such a burst of activity while moving its contents along that it telescopes into the segment ahead of it. If this segment gets "stuck," there is serious trouble. Needless to say, the vaccine was discontinued later in the same year it was approved. Two new vaccines appeared in 2006. The oral vaccine currently is incorporated into the "routine" infant immunization schedule, and has been approved by the World Health Organization (WHO) for a mass vaccination program in South Africa and Malawi. It appears to be greatly reducing the incidence of this diarrhea illness there. If this vaccine continues to be proven safe, I can approve its use in areas that have poor medical facilities and poor hygiene, but I see no general need for it in this country.

The pneumococcal vaccine was introduced in the year 2000. It was developed to provide immunity to a bacterium, *Streptococcus pneumoniae* (its older name is simply pneumococcus). It is easy to see "pneumonia" in the name. It is a cause of a particular type of pneumonia and also of middle ear infections—a more frequent pediatric problem—and of much more serious, invasive diseases such as meningitis or sepsis (infection in the bloodstream).

Since most bouts of pneumonia are not due to this organism, it bothers me that seniors are admonished to get their "pneumonia" shot. Pneumococci, meningococci and *H. influenzae* are part of a class of bacteria that contain a polysaccharide in their cell membranes. Polysaccharide vaccines (see Hib) don't stimulate a good immune response in children younger than two or three years of age. So that first vaccine was a "conjugated" vaccine but contained only seven different strains of pneumococci (known as the pneumococcal 7-valent conjugate vaccine). By 2003 it was highly touted. By April of 2007 it was reported in *Medscape* that the most common bacterial isolates (obtained from people in the community) were species *not* contained in the vaccine. By September 2010 it was found that the 7-valent vaccine was facilitating acquisition of a serotype not in the vaccine (serotype 19A) that was causing serious invasive disease such as empyema (an infection in the covering of the pleura that requires surgical intervention). A new 13-valent vaccine was promptly developed. Currently there is even a 23-valent vaccine available.

ZINC, VITAMIN D FIGHT PNEUMONIA IN BABIES AND TODDLERS

In a double-blind, randomized, placebo-controlled clinical trial, 352 children with severe pneumonia, aged six to fifty-nine months, were given zinc supplements. Children one year or older were given 20 mg of zinc, and those below twelve months were given 10 mg. Death rate in the placebo group was 12 percent, but only 4 percent in the zinc supplement group. The authors add that among HIV-infected children, over a quarter of the no-zinc group died, and *none* of the zinc-supplemented HIV children died. They concluded that "zinc supplementation in these children significantly decreased case fatality."[1]

More good news: Researchers report that vitamin D supplementation will reduce the risk of repeat pneumonia episodes. Two hundred and twenty-four children (one to thirty-six months of age) received 100,000 international units (IU) of vitamin D. "The risk of a repeat episode of pneumonia within 90 days of supplementation was lower . . . [and] children in the vitamin D_3 group survived longer without experiencing a repeat episode."[2]

There is also evidence that higher vitamin D levels reduced influenza and pneumonia fatalities during the great 1918–1919 pandemic, when millions died. The authors write, for the benefit of physicians wanting to know the precise biochemical mechanism, "Vitamin D upregulates production of human cathelicidin, LL-37, which has both antimicrobial and antiendotoxin activities. Vitamin D also reduces the production of proinflammatory cytokines, which could also explain some of the benefit of vitamin D since H1N1 infection gives rise to a cytokine storm."[3] Talk about this with your pediatrician. This article illustrates the fact that "even your average doctor" might only get the gist of what is stated and not the particulars. He or she has to rely on the honesty and expertise of the source, and see if it fits with what is considered general medical knowledge.

References

1. Srinivasan, M. G., G. Ndeezi, C. K. Mboijana, et al. "Zinc Adjunct Therapy Reduces Case Fatality in Severe Childhood Pneumonia: A Randomized Double Blind Placebo-Controlled Trial." *BMC Med* 10 (Feb 8, 2012):14.

2. Manaseki-Holland, S., G. Qader, M. Isaq Masher, et al. "Effects of Vitamin D Supplementation to Children Diagnosed with Pneumonia in Kabul: A Randomised Controlled Trial." *Trop Med Int Health* (15(10) (Oct 2010): 1148–1155.

3. Grant, W. B., E. Giovannucci. "The Possible Roles of Solar Ultraviolet-B Radiation and Vitamin D in Reducing Case-Fatality Rates from the 1918–1919 Influenza Pandemic in the United States. *Dermatoendocrinol* 1(4) (Jul 2009):215–219.

The human spleen is able to sequester these pneumococci bacteria from the bloodstream. Individuals must be super careful about infection with any of these bacteria if their spleen has been removed or if it functions poorly due to certain disorders, such as sickle cell anemia, or if their immune system is subpar. They should be immunized with the latest vaccine. They will likely also be subjected to "unnecessary" antibiotic treatment, since once a seemingly minor infection gets underway, it rapidly becomes deadly. But for a normal infant, I believe that continuing to give three shots of this vaccine by six months could provide more harm than help for the infant immune system.

A hepatitis A vaccine has been available since 1995. Hepatitis A virus infection is the Public Health poster child for diseases spread by the fecal-oral route. To avoid it, *wash your hands* after going to the bathroom. Travelers south of the border do well in being very careful of what they eat or drink. Bottling facilities provide safe beverages, and fruit should be peeled. Like every other illness, there are a few severe cases among the majority of not-so-bad cases. Many escape the appearance of jaundice (the telltale sign is yellow skin and whites of eyes). Since hygiene measures can keep adults free of disease, even in occupations that would relate to high exposure, routine vaccination is not recommended. It is difficult for me to understand why the AAP's immunization schedule recommends two shots for children between twelve and eighteen months of age, with six months in between. If my math is correct, this would mean at twelve months, and again at eighteen months. This is better than if the recommendation was for starting at birth, as it is for the hepatitis B vaccination; but I still categorically give this vaccination a thumbs-down rating for infants. Exceptions would involve situations of unusual and intense exposure, in which hygienic measures can't be followed—such as when no potable water is available.

Schedules include meningococcal vaccine to be given between two and six years of age. Meninigococcal meningitis is typically the type of meningitis that occurs when people are living in crowded conditions and under stress. And there are menigococcal infections other than meningitis that are serious but rare. It has always been a difficult problem for the military, where people live under stress in close quarters. Now, vaccine promoters are promoting the idea that this is what college life is like. Many colleges demand that incoming students be vaccinated. A current television advertisement from the meningococcal vaccine manufacturers shows a young man with missing distal extremities because they required amputation. Very rarely, infection from this bacterium causes a blood-borne condition (septicemia) that obliterates the small arteries at the ends of extremities. The conveyed message was: "I am lucky to be alive, but don't let this horrible thing happen to you. Get the vaccine."

I have seen only one case of meningitis due to this organism in my pediatric practice. This four-year-old did well with treatment and had no residual problems from the disease. But watch out now: It seems our FDA can always come up with powerful reasons to support their approval of new vaccines. In April of 2011, a vaccine to prevent invasive meningococcal disease in infants (given at nine months of age) was approved. The FDA states that the highest *rate* of meningococcal disease in children occurs in individuals under one year of age. There is no statement of absolute numbers. I suspect it is a very low number. Again, unless your infant mingles on a day-to-day basis with many other infants, I would feel that this vaccine would not be necessary. Your pediatrician should provide you with the actual incidence of meningococcal disease in infants.

The Question of Autism and Immunizations

There is another problem concerning infants receiving immunizations, particularly the MMR vaccine—is it a cause of autism or the broader "autism spectrum" disease? This has become a heated controversy, full of emotional content. MMR was one of the first vaccines to use thimerosal as a preservative. Thimerosal contains nearly 50 percent ethylmercury, a form of mercury known to be toxic to the nervous system. The immature nervous system is much more susceptible to damage from such chemicals. The vaccine industry, with support from the FDA, has staunchly denied any connection between this preservative and autism or the more inclusive "autism spectrum disease." In spite of this stance, the AAP in its 1999 *Handbook of Pediatric Environmental Health,* distributed to all pediatricians, stated that even though there is no *proof* of this relationship, infants receiving thimerosal-containing vaccines during the early months of life *could* be exposed to more mercury than recommended by federal guidelines. In July 1999 they *asked* manufacturers to eliminate or *reduce* the mercury content of vaccines. The "Danish study," started in 2002, was said by vaccine proponents to have laid to rest any question of the association of autism to thimerosal in vaccines. The United States Centers for Disease Control and Prevention (CDC) substantially agrees.[7] This controversy is ongoing. We question why such a study had to be done in Denmark, and even when it was, why an author had ties to the vaccination industry such that the study's objectivity was being publicly questioned.[8]

MERCURY IN MEDICINE AND DENTISTRY

One of the common remedies of the eighteenth and nineteenth centuries was mercury. Mercury is well known today to be a toxic heavy metal, the very vapors of which are dangerous. Any junior-high science teacher knows this (and I, AWS, was one), and has in the lab classroom a mercury clean-up kit for immediate, safe isolation of any spill, no matter how small. No longer will grade-school friends be allowed to play with "quicksilver," elemental mercury's common name. No longer may anyone roll the heavy, cold, shiny liquid about in their hands and try to coat pennies with it. It is too dangerous.

Yet in the not-too-far past, mercury, often as the drug calomel, was administered to countless innocent and trusting patients, not by medicine show quacks but by the family doctor. Well, we can dismiss the dark ages of medicine as over and done with, right? Wrong. Mercury, making up over half of a so-called "silver" amalgam dental filling, is still placed into the living bone tissue of adults and children, where it may well stay—twenty-four hours a day, seven days a week—for ten years or more. Some of my mercury amalgam fillings lasted me from childhood into fatherhood. If a science teacher encouraged a thirteen-year-old to put mercury into his mouth, it would be gross negligence bordering on criminal. Dentists have done it every day, for over a hundred years.

Enough is enough. Insist on white composite fillings. They are mercury-free, last a long time, and hopefully, are the only form of cavity restorations that your dentist will offer you.

Adjuvants in Vaccines

Attention has been brought only recently to the problem of adjuvants in vaccines. Adjuvants are added pharmacological agents designed to boost the immune response to a vaccine. They do it by creating inflammation, which activates the immune system much the way fever does. Aluminum was one of the early adjuvants, which could explain why a reaction of heat and pain at the injection site was so common. At that time, we were told nothing about such products. We must question whether promoting inflammation as a legitimate means of enhancing an immune response is a good idea, since inflammation is regarded as a factor in almost every chronic disease.

TOO MANY SHOTS, AND WAY TOO SOON

By the time an infant reaches his or her first birthday, if current recommendations are followed, he or she will have been injected with thirty-five antigens and, depending on the combinations, from sixteen to twenty-three shots. The harm is much more than inflicting pain, creating inflamed sites of injection, or even production of severe, nervous system insults—tangible effects that are rare. We are bound to create problems by bombarding the infant's immature immune system and nervous system with multiple vaccinations that contain adjuvants as well as preservatives, also of unproven safety. The vaccine industry asks for proof that vaccines create problems. It is difficult to fix blame on a single cause when there are multiple factors that can contribute to mental or behavioral problems. Immune responses to vaccines are individually based, depending on the person's immune health, and must be considered that way. One shoe size does *not* fit all. Nor can the industry "prove" that there is *no* harm inflicted. What is being denied and not opened to fair scrutiny is that immature immune and nervous systems are being attacked by these many vaccinations. Infants are being subjected to more than they can handle.

We should start the use of some of these vaccines when the infants are somewhat older and their immune systems are further along the road to maturity. We should also revert to giving fewer "combined" shots in early infancy. We need to remind vaccine manufacturers of their past miscalculations and the lack of studies proving safety and efficacy. Pressure must be applied to the FDA to show more transparency in their methods of evaluating and accepting studies devised by the industry itself. Many advocate an independent body be established to do this work.

I have little hope that it will happen in the U.S. But an orthomolecular medicine practitioner in Japan, Atsuo Yanagisawa, M.D., Ph.D., tells me that Japan has a two-tiered immunization system. Some vaccines are mandatory; many are voluntary. And they are started at a later age (usually after two years of age). This model should be honestly studied. Dr. Yanagisawa had no data suggesting a relationship between autism spectrum disorder (ASD) and the MMR vaccination, because ASD is rare in Japan. Hmmm.

A pediatric neurologist I (RKC) heard speak at a meeting of pediatricians had an interesting theory that was somewhat "tongue in cheek." He said that a normal, healthy toddler's neurological wiring was all mixed up. "They see with their hands—'Let me see that'—as they grab something out of your hands. They hear with their eyes: you might as well be talking to a wall if you don't have eye contact with a toddler." Interesting, that such eye contact is missing in autistic children and is practiced in therapy sessions with them.

NO FREEDOM OF CHOICE

Perhaps the biggest change needed in the current handling of vaccinations is eliminating the mandates by medical authorities that disallow parental choice, even well-informed choice. Vaccine manufacturers have had their way with legislators. It is an unconscionable act to make the mother of a newborn sign a consent form so her infant will receive its first (unnecessary) hepatitis B shot while the child is still in the newborn nursery. Unfortunately, once health officials accept recommendations by certain authoritative medical associations, such as the AAP, regulations and enforcement procedures follow. These vary from state to state and can easily get out of hand. Creators of regulations need to be better informed and not blindly follow the recommendations of "medical authorities." We believe that informed parents should never be forced to inflict their infants with a vaccine they do not want. We further assert that exemptions from specific vaccines can often be made after a discussion with an understanding and well-informed doctor, that can still comply with local regulations.

In theory, that is possible. The practical truth is that it is difficult to prove to a medical doctor that your children specifically will suffer a great health risk by being vaccinated. Fear of a possible allergic reaction to the shot(s) would be a valid argument. Great susceptibility to side effects or a pre-existing high-risk condition could also be given as reasons. This is hard to implement; most physicians will side with orthodoxy and public health policy.

Even if your doctor did exempt you, it is very probable that he or she will be called on the carpet by the authorities to defend why the child shouldn't be vaccinated. This approach puts the burden of proof on both you and the doctor, and will only be as strong as the weaker link. When faced with losing a medical license that the doctor worked twelve years to get, guess who the weaker link likely will be?

Religious Freedom

A more radical way of getting around vaccination regulations is also the simpler way: Take a religious exception to vaccination on spiritual grounds. This is constitutionally valid; remember that the First Amendment guarantees freedom of religion.

There are two parallel religious avenues to consider, and I (AWS) have used them both. First, you can join a religious group that holds vaccinations in disfavor. If this is unacceptable or impractical, you can actually start a church organization that believes vaccinations are morally wrong. Such a church may certainly "forbid any serum, vaccine, foreign, unnatural, or chemical substance of any nature to be injected or ingested into a church member's body for any avowed medical purpose whatsoever."

LANDMARK ANTI-VACCINATION DECISION IN NEW YORK

In many states including New York, it has always been relatively simple to attend school without any shots at all . . . if you have a religious exemption. But what about parents of children that are already partially immunized, and then change their mind? They have been often been denied a religious exemption due to health department or school officials' claims that their religious beliefs are not "sincerely held," since they have already had vaccinations prior to their new request for religious exemption.

In January 2002, U.S. District Court Judge Michael A. Telesca wrote an important precedent-setting decision: "This court may not pass on the wisdom of belief, nor on the manner upon which she came to hold that belief, provided that she maintains a sincere and genuine religious objection to immunization." In other words, once a person decides that they do not want any more shots for reasons of religious conscience their decision is valid even if they previously had their child immunized.

The case is also important because the family in question was devoutly Roman Catholic. The Vatican is not opposed to vaccination. This decision allows individual members of a mainstream church organization to hold personal spiritual beliefs in addition to their church's official doctrine.

What's more, the family had previously sought, and been denied, a medical exemption from vaccination. The judge's ruling renders this point irrelevant.

Reference

Tokasz, J. "Judge Forces School to Accept Girl." *Democrat and Chronicle* Rochester, NY (Jan 31, 2002):B1.

Your second approach option depends on your state's laws. Many states, such as New York, where I (AWS) live, no longer require a designated church affiliation because to do so would probably be unconstitutional. Instead, parents or guardians must hold "genuine and sincere religious beliefs" that are contrary to vaccination. This means that a simple affidavit stating those beliefs in one or two sentences may suffice. An affidavit is as simple as having both parents sign a very short statement in the presence of a notary public. Your bank or town clerk will likely notarize for no charge.

You are still not home free. Taking a religious exemption to shots means you have to make an all-or-none decision. You cannot religiously object to some shots and not to others. That is why targeted medical exemption, as previously described by Dr. Campbell, is preferred. It is also nearly impossible to obtain, or to keep when obtained. Until our nation allows physicians and parents to make the decision as to exactly which shots they want, you are stuck with these extremes.

CHAPTER 3

PROBLEMS
OR JUST QUESTIONS?

I am going to anticipate, by thinking back to what got *my* attention as a new father, those conditions your child may experience that would prompt your curiosity and require reassuring answers. A newborn, in particular, can exhibit lots of unique conditions that are unfamiliar to new parents.

THE SKIN

We will start with skin conditions. Many of these are transient, so they can be described easily and then dismissed—simply noted during the well baby checkup. Not to worry! We will go from the transient and less worrisome to the more problematic conditions.

Skin Problems in New Infants

Many skin conditions are typical in new infants, while some are more common in older infants. We will discuss both. Many of these problems can usually be easily controlled—and as you will see, some are not really "problems" at all.

Vernix Caseosa

If a just-new mother is alert enough, she might see her newborn covered with a white substance that resembles a "night cream" or a heavy-duty lotion. The substance's official name is *vernix caseosa* due to its cheesy consistency. It is made up of skin oils and shed epithelial cells. In some birthing centers, the baby is immediately whisked off to be "cleaned up." So mother's quick assessment causes her to ask, "What on earth is that?" This covering might not look appropriate for a beautiful new baby, but it is there for a good reason. The fatty coating is protective for the fetus who is being constantly bathed in amniotic fluid, in much the same way as lanolin is used to cover and protect the body of a "channel swimmer." It has a mild antibacterial property, which is a real asset for a baby being born in less than desirable (not sterile) conditions (as babies were through most of history and even today, in a third-world country).

Erythema Toxicum

Erythema toxicum means "red spots or bumps suspected of being due to some toxin." The medical name is vague because the nature of the toxin is not known. I think it is an allergen derived when the fetus swallows amniotic fluid while in the womb—fluid from mother could contain particles of mother's allergens.

This rash can have a diverse appearance, anywhere from papules (bumps) to splotches. It peaks in two days and doesn't last, which fits in with my thought of the baby having had exposure and then escaping from some allergen.

Sebaceous Hyperplasia

This term refers to an "overproduction of the sebaceous glands," which secrete an oily substance under the skin. Little whiteheads appear over the face and forehead, as if the final exit of the material is blocked at the surface. Larger whiteheads are given the name "milia." The condition is probably due to transient maternal hormone levels and will disappear in a few weeks.

Salmon Patch

Salmon patch is a pink, flat spot on the forehead or, more commonly, on the nape of the neck—what pediatricians call a "stork bite." These spots can persist for several months. One on the face, located between the eyes and extending upwards, is often called a "flame nevus," due to its shape. Either one will eventually fade. Those on the nape will be covered with hair. Both will grow more highly colored with crying.

Mongolian Spots

Mongolian spots are well demarcated and usually occur over the sacrum and buttocks. They are very common in black babies, less so in white. Although they are quite noticeable, be assured that they will eventually fade away. They will not mar the infant's beauty given that they are in the diaper area. No one seems to know how they got the moniker Mongolian (or Mongol) spots. They don't form in just Mongolians, and they are much larger than your average "spot." A baby will have only one large spot—not spots.

As an aside: I served with a team of social workers who were investigating infants suspected of being victims of an abusive parent. It soon became apparent that they needed more training, as some regarded Mongol spots as bruises and a "thrush" diaper rash (discussed next) as a sign of parental neglect.

Diaper Rash

Diaper rash may be considered a form of contact dermatitis caused by laundry soaps or bath soaps, or a rash superimposed on skin that is constantly wet or subjected to ammonia formed in the diaper. If the latter, your nose can make the diagnosis. It doesn't occur in the immediate newborn period because its presence depends on the intestinal flora. The newborn's gut is essentially sterile; so it doesn't contain bacteria capable of chemically splitting the urea of urine into ammonia. (Ammonia and urea are used as nitrogen sources in commercial fertilizers. Soil bacteria reduce either one to nitrogen, much the same as intestinal bacteria convert the urea in urine to ammonia.)

Breast milk encourages the development of beneficial bacterial intestinal flora that crowd out the common bacteria that have this enzymatic ability to form ammonia. So, breast-fed babies do better in this respect. Once established, the ammonia-forming bacteria in the formula-fed baby tend to persist and will worsen when new foods are added. In more severe instances, blisters form in the area. The wet, macerated skin then invites a secondary yeast (monilial or *Candida*) infection.

A monilial rash can look angry and itch. It can cover most of the diaper area with a rose-colored, flat rash that resists the common treatment of keeping the area dry and clean—which is applicable for all forms of diaper dermatitis. The pros and cons of disposable versus cloth diapers should be considered.

Cloth diapers. If cloth diapers are used, it may be helpful to use something as simple as vinegar (a weak acid) in the diaper pail to neutralize the ammonia. You do not need more than a splash or two, either cider or white vinegar will work fine. Avoid plastic pants, which hold in moisture, with either type of diaper. Instead, place the baby *on* a diaper, without pinning it, for some periods during the day. Change the diaper often. If "water-proofing" is needed, a zinc oxide or other heavy ointment can be used, but only on dry skin (don't seal in moisture). You can also use vitamin E, but again, only on dry skin. Most vitamin E is in an oil form, and oil and water do not mix on babies' bottoms any better than they do in salad dressing.

Disposable Diapers. Same basic approach as above, but without the diaper pail. Isn't that one of the main reasons why you chose them, anyhow? Hmm?

Oral thrush, which manifests as white areas on the inner surface of the cheeks, roof of mouth, and tongue, will need treatment, and is proof that the intestinal tract is supporting an overgrowth of yeast. A diaper-area rash due to monilial (Candida) infection can be treated with an antifungal cream. Oral thrush might require its own topical treatment or even systemic treatment with medication. Before taking that step, there is a simple remedy to try first: yogurt. Yogurt contains probiotic (good) bacteria that help inhibit intestinal fungal/yeast overgrowths. The friendly microorganisms in yogurt inhibit bad bacteria in the digestive tract, reduce excess alkalinity, and also improve the baby's immune system as part of the bargain. Even a breastfeeding baby can be given a tiny amount of plain yogurt. We're talking a fraction of a teaspoon here. Mom can even coat the nipple with yogurt, and even that will do the trick. A thimbleful of yogurt has literally billions of helpful microorganisms. Sounds offbeat, perhaps but consider this: I (AWS) had a friend with a baby with diaper rash from knees to navel. It was severe and medication was not doing much, if anything, to alleviate it. The parents started externally coating the affected area of the infant's skin with room-temperature plain yogurt. Really. And it worked very well for them: We are talking relief overnight and resolution in just a few days. And that was one wicked case of diaper rash, let me tell you. Internally and/or externally, Lactobacillus- and *Bifidobacterium infantis* can really help fight monilial and other fungal bugs.

Skin Problems in Older Infants

As the infant gets older, many of the skin conditions related to very early infancy disappear or decrease in frequency and severity. New issues may begin to appear at this time.

Cradle Cap

Cradle cap in an older infant is well named. Occasionally, in the dry form, it appears almost like dandruff—yellowish flakes that can be gently combed out. Usually it forms more greasy flakes that consolidate and can not be easily removed. The treatment is frequent shampooing. Precede the shampoo with the application of baby oil (mineral oil), dabbed on with a cotton ball, to the entire stubborn area of the scalp, to attempt to free up the scales. If the process gets ahead of you, be content with whittling away at the problem a little at a time. Once it is clear, it is usually easy to keep clear.

Seborrhea

Seborrhea (or seborrheic dermatitis) comes on later still; cradle cap is a mild, more restricted variant. It can occur any time from infancy into full adulthood. Besides its presence in the scalp, seborrhea can be seen as dry yellowish scales in the eyebrows, ears, and sides of nose, accompanied with red skin folds. If the scales are thick there is redness underneath, and it can itch a little and resemble mild eczema. An adult is usually prescribed an antidandruff (antiseborrheic) shampoo. After looking at the numerous chemicals in these shampoos, labeled as "inactive ingredients," I have never felt comfortable in prescribing this treatment for infants. A baby shampoo should suffice. I have prescribed B vitamins when the simple treatments of avoiding harsh soaps or hot water bathing is not sufficient.

As a pediatric resident in training, I (RKC) was privileged to witness a very rare case of Leiner disease. This newborn was literally covered with seborrheic scales from head to toe. This nearly complete covering created a circumstance that had to be corrected promptly, because the scales did not permit sweat to make it all the way to the surface of the baby's body, nor did they allow for good heat disbursement. Fortunately, when I called my doctor mentor, he not only knew what I was dealing with but also had just happened to have learned of the solution—biotin, one of the B vitamins. *And* he just happened to have a couple of vials of biotin solution, suitable for injection, on hand. A courier negotiated the fifty-mile road trip with this precious stuff, which I gave immediately. The result was truly miraculous. In just a few days, most of the scaliness was gone. Biotin is part of an enzyme that is a carrier of carbon dioxide, so it is involved with essential carboxylation reactions needed by our bodies. We usually get enough biotin from our diet so as not to allow anything as severe as this case.

Some feel that biotin is hardly a vitamin, meaning that it must be derived from a nutritional source, since we can get most of what we need from synthesis by our bacterial intestinal flora. With no intestinal flora in the newborn to manufacture it, there must have been something that blocked the effectiveness of the enzyme contained in the maternal blood passed on to the infant. A big dose of biotin broke through the blockade. Biotin is one of the B complex vitamins. I have helped many seborrhea (seborrheic dermatitis) sufferers by suggesting an inexpensive B50 preparation. This fills their biotin need and adds many extra dividends.

Eczema

Eczema is discussed in the "Allergy Problems" section. I mention it here because seborrheic dermatitis can have an inflammatory element that may cause itching, and an angry appearance that resembles eczema.

THE HEAD

Head shape and other evidence that a relatively big head had to squeeze through the birth canal are immediately apparent. If we consider these dimensions, we might say, "It can't be done." Contemplate the amazing way that it *is* done. The newborn's skull is not fixed in size. That comes later in normal development. There are several divisions, called sutures, among the different bones that make up the skull. One runs "north-south" along the top of the skull, a major one runs "east-west," and another "east-west" suture is closer to the back of the head. These different plates of bone are not complete, and they form spaces (soft spots or fontanels) where they butt up against one another—one large one near the front of the skull with a smaller one rearward. The necessary reduction in size during birth comes about by some overlapping of these soft bones at the sutures and crowding of the open spaces. A pretty clever arrangement, yes?

Head Distortion, Edemas, and Hematomas

The scalp and head can be distorted by the shearing forces of birth. These forces can also cause a firm "knot" of edema fluid (like a "hickey") or even of the covering of the bone, which can tear small blood vessels and cause an escape of blood—a hematoma. The distortions of head shape and the edema-fluid knots normally clear in a few days, while the hematoma might take weeks. In a few days the hematoma will be soft in the middle and firm around the periphery. When the free blood finally liquefies, the hematoma seems to "deflate" overnight. An interesting side effect of this is the appearance of some yellowing of the skin due to bilirubin, a natural breakdown product of blood as it is taken up by the bloodstream. This, too, soon fades.

GASTROINTESTINAL "THINGS"

A newborn's first bowel movements are very (shall we say) different. Fetuses swallow the amniotic fluid they are suspended in. The entire stomach and intestinal tract "tune up," as it were, in preparation for life in the outside world. A baby undergoing stress during the birthing process can actually have a bowel movement that mingles with the amniotic fluid, turning it dark. The first dark stool, of a rather tarry consistency, is called meconium. Meconium is formed from sloughed-off cells of the intestinal tract and other swallowed material. Bile is being excreted into the intestinal tract and plays a part in creating the dark, tarry stuff due to the breakdown of old fetal red cells. (All red blood cells live only so long and are broken down and replenished in a normal cycle.) This meconium is usually passed within the first twenty-four hours after birth.

Hemoglobin is the iron-containing protein in red blood cells that enables the exchange of oxygen and carbon dioxide in the various tissues of our body. Myoglobin is the protein that performs this same function at the other end of the exchange (in the muscle tissues). Depending on the oxygen and carbon dioxide levels in the blood at any one time, these "smart" substances know just how to work. The fetal heart is designed so that oxygenated blood from mother's circulation won't be sent into the fetal, nonfunctioning, lungs. For this reason the fetus has its own brand of hemoglobin, which uses different levels of oxygenation than will be present once the baby starts to breathe on its own. In the newborn period there is a rapid transition from fetal hemoglobin to adult hemoglobin, which accelerates bilirubin production as the fetal hemoglobin breaks down. Also, with the infant's new circulation system activating, excess blood volume is rapidly reduced, resulting in higher bilirubin levels. The newborn liver can't keep with the pace of converting bilirubin into bile for excretion. All this leads to jaundice, which, to some degree, occurs in over 50 percent of normal newborns. In addition to the skin having a yellow cast to it, there can be rare, more serious, consequences. Fortunately, if problems do develop, they become apparent while the newborn is still in the hospital under observation. This supports the argument for keeping the infant in the hospital for a *reasonable* length of time, where a close watch can be kept on the rapidity of the rise in bilirubin and the absolute high levels that could be dangerous. If a newborn is growing moderately jaundiced, he or she will likely be put under a bank of lights (bilirubin lights). These beam on a large area of exposed skin and use the proper light spectrum that causes a breakdown of bilirubin. This treatment discovery has been a blessing, because it takes the place of much more tedious means of flushing bilirubin from the blood—the exchange transfusion. Early hospital discharge requires that mother be responsible for looking out for any noted increase in the yellow skin color and reporting to her doctor—a rare condition these days, but one that must be evaluated.

The "Diapered End"

The transitional stools that follow about three or four days after milk feedings start are greenish brown, reflecting the excess of bilirubin. After another three or four days the stools are more consistently normal infant stools. Odor and consistency depend on the establishment of the intestinal flora. A good intestinal flora is more easily established in a breast-fed baby. There is a wide variation in the number of stools per day for a normal baby, depending on the frequency of feedings and the amount per feeding; usually there are three to five per day by the end of the first week. Occasionally, a normal baby will have no stool at all for an entire day, while another baby may have as many as six or seven a day once feeding is established—especially with a breast-fed baby. Not to worry about these extremes if there is no sign of abdominal distension along with real fussiness.

Spitting Up

It is a common thing for babies to spit up a bit after feeding. Successful burping is a big help. As much as possible strive for a calm atmosphere at feeding time. Formula-fed babies have a worse time with spitting up than breast-fed babies, probably because it is harder to regulate the speed of feeding. Surely, a baby who gulps air as he or she feeds too eagerly is more apt to spit up. With gravity feed, an upside-down bottle should release only about a drop per second. (A blind, unpierced, bottle nipple can be customized with a hot needle.)

Sooner or later all "feeders" will be baptized with the white, sour stuff as they hold the baby after feeding. Spitting can become a problem when large amounts of formula are spit up. In addition to trying the calming methods (see the colic chapter), it might be necessary to prop the infant up for a time after feeding. I used to suggest thickened feedings—adding cereal to the formula given through a "sloppy" nipple with a bigger hole. But this greatly altered the sucking experience. I suspect that when this inconvenient treatment didn't seem to work and because it was so messy, it was abandoned and renewed effort was made trying the alternatives. There has been a tendency for pediatricians to treat heavy spitting with a medicine that supposedly allows a better balance of action between the stomach valve (between the stomach and the intestinal tract) and the valve between the stomach and the esophagus. There are too many drawbacks to treating gastroesophageal reflux (GER) with medicines. Keep it simple; call it old-fashioned "spitting up." First try the simple, harmless solutions. (It is apparent to me that the purpose of pining a diagnosis of GER on an infant who, like many, has nothing more seriously wrong other than being messy, is to promote the sale of acid-stopping drugs. Stomach acid is *essential* for normal digestion and assimilation of trace minerals. If "spit-up" lacks the sour smell, something *is* drastically wrong. The current description of, and treatment for, GER in infants is nearly identical of what I have described. Even thickened feedings are back in vogue. It is often stated that the condition is usually over after the first few months of life. We should not assume that infants, who are more readily upset with drugs, are just little adults who have an appetite for medicines.

Umbilical Hernia

There is an opening in the central "seam" of the abdomen that the umbilical cord goes through. After the cord is cut and the stump of it dries and sloughs off, the skin closes over to form the belly button, but the opening can remain. In some infants crying can produce bulging that can be seen above the belly button and a considerable way up this middle seam. The stomach muscle's edges can be easily felt. The round opening of the hernia itself can measure an inch or more. If it is larger, it will be obvious that a loop of intestine is pushing through. It can easily be pushed back (reduced). No one is certain whether intervention by taping the bands of abdominal muscles together is effective for this condition, which somehow seems to resolve on its own. A small umbilical hernia causes no harm.

CONCLUSION

What we have described in this chapter are not abnormalities, just variations of normal—part of the ballgame. A few zits don't detract from the overall beauty and wonder of a newborn!

CHAPTER 4

COLIC AND DIARRHEA

New parents often face two common, troublesome issues: diarrhea and colic. Both cause great distress and discomfort for the child as well as his or her parents—including many hours of lost sleep and frustration. Although both have similar fallout, it is important to note that they are not similar in cause: One is a digestive issue and one is an illness that can be very serious.

COLIC

Everyone knows what diarrhea is, but what do we mean by colic? The classic definition is that colic is a condition in infants characterized by loud and prolonged crying for which no physiological or other cause has been found. *Dorland's Medical Dictionary* has the usual medical mumbo-jumbo: "Acute abdominal pain, characteristically, intermittent visceral pain with fluctuating corresponding smooth muscle peristalsis." Loud and prolonged crying—true. But I disagree with "no cause has been found." The translation of the medical definition boils down to "a severe belly ache with periods of cramping." From these definitions, we gain a bit of an idea of what is going on with the infant, but little of the effect of the infant's distress on its mother and the rest of the household.

As for myself, I am sure that I can never fully appreciate how exhausting, physically as well as mentally, the process must be. Add to that even just a touch of anxiety about all the new tasks and responsibilities that are thrust upon a new mother. Some sort of an instinctual protection program must kick in for all mammalian mothers that modulates these destructive forces, or survival for either mother or infant would be tough to achieve. We "strong" men have to truly admire the tremendous strength of mothers. Even a thoughtful, vigorous dad has a tough time coping with sleep interruption. Nowadays it seems that hospitals or birthing centers want mother and baby discharged as soon as possible, as if teaching both to swim by throwing them into the water. One of the ways to gain strength to deal with motherhood is to enjoy restorative sleep. Cruel joke, that. If her newborn is sleeping quietly, is she still breathing? If she is crying, is it from hunger, a wet diaper, or some other cause of discomfort? Mom has to wake herself up enough to make a decision—let it go and hope crying goes away, or get up and take a look, or nudge hubby and let him get up. Parents are "Sleepless in Seattle" and every other city, too.

There is nothing more disturbing, not just of sleep, but of one's very soul, than that loud and prolonged crying from a precious newborn. Something has to be done, or sleep deprivation takes its toll on the psyche as well as the body. We know, deep down, that the baby is not crying just to disturb us, but we can't help wonder why he or she stubbornly resists all attempts to provide comfort as we act out of love. In time, these negative effects on thought processes can turn feelings of love into resentment. Gentle jiggling done by an exhausted caregiver might become too intense—and endanger both lives. We must not allow this faulty interaction due to exhaustion and frustration to go this far.

What to Do

Instead of going further into the dynamics and dire consequences of doing nothing, let's get to the good part: The problem *can* be remedied. We *can* get our cuddly baby back. Without referring to an exacting clinical description, most parents will pinpoint what prompts their baby to cry so persistently and forcibly. The infant is saying, "I am in pain. Do something." He (we'll use the "generic" gender in this instance) draws up his legs and has a tense abdomen that when gently thumped reveals that he is full of gas that he can neither burp nor pass from the other end. Rocking, patting, offering more feeding (or a so-called pacifier), listening to soothing singing, a ride in the car, getting others to give it a go with their method of soothing—nothing does the trick. (Any of these age-old remedies should be questioned, due to individual differences in the infant and their particular situation. Some hypersensitive infants consider any of the "action" solutions as adding to their "stimulation package." We like to express love to our dog friends by patting them on the head, but I don't think all dogs like that. I know *I* don't.) It is obvious that peace will not come until that gas leaves. So why won't it leave?

We can get into the exceptions to the rule later, but for the most part gas (or just plain gulped air) is trapped at either end by sphincters (ring-like valves) held tightly closed by tension. The good thing about a colicky baby is that he is overly alert (smart), making him overly sensitive to his surroundings. A day might go well until around four in the afternoon, at which time he has had it with all the stimuli and begins to tune up. He feeds like it might be his only feeding until morning. He can be heard to gulp and swallow, not just the feeding, but quantities of air. Burping doesn't get the desired result. If soothing methods are successful enough to enable putting him down in the crib, there still is more squirming and more reaction to noises and other sensory stimuli than usual. Then sincere crying begins. The swallowed air has made its way from the stomach into the small intestine, which produces pain when distended. We adults, who have suffered an intestinal upset, know what that is like. It is almost a blessing to have diarrhea begin when it gives relief of the distension and the accompanying severe bellyache. The cycle of more distension, more pain, more crying, and more swallowed air must be broken. Some way must be found that provides enough comfort to the infant to allow relaxation of the sphincters.

One inexpert description of colic states that contrary to the belief that babies cry from swallowed air, x-ray studies reveal that when babies start wailing they have less air trapped in their stomachs than they do when the colic is over. The study's timing with x-rays was out of synch. It is only when the air leaves the stomach and enters the small intestine that the "wailing" begins. When the crying is over, the gas has exited by the back door.

Swaddling

The answer is, in large part, found in swaddling. It worked for baby Jesus. And I'll bet Moses' mother swaddled him, preparing him for a *quiet* journey to a safe place down the Nile. A straitjacket isn't placed on an out-of-control, raging person as a means of punishment, but to break the cycle of self-stimulation caused by the wild movement. A dog going crazy on the Fourth of July is better off in a quiet, darkened room away from stimulation. The more an overly stimulated infant flails arms and legs about, the more "out of it" he or she becomes.

It would be nice to enclose a video that showed proper swaddling technique with this book, but let's attempt to provide some written instruction:

1. Lay out a lightweight receiving blanket. Place the baby on its back catty-corner to the blanket (head and feet towards corners). Fold the top corner down so that the top edge is even with the baby's shoulders (head protruding).

2. Put an arm at a 45-degree angle next to the body and tuck in the material that lies above the arm.

3. Take the outside corner of the blanket on the same side as the arm in step 2 and pull it across the body. Tuck it in under the baby's back on the other side of the body so that the arm ends up folded across the body, the forearm perpendicular to the body.

4. Repeat steps 2 and 3 with the second arm, making sure that the corners are tucked in securely (this may require pinning).

5. Pick him up and put his back to your chest with your arms supporting him under his knees.

You can usually see a look of contentment, or "wha' happened," as a result of finding comfort. And you should then be able to transfer him into a slightly tilted back portable infant car seat (contour chair position) that will duplicate what you accomplished.

Hospital and residency training ill equips one for the *practice* of pediatrics. True education begins when surrounded by experienced doctors and nurses where real practice begins. I was fortunate when starting my pediatric practice to partner with a very intelligent and creative pediatrician, John C. Wilcox. He taught me the swaddling technique I just described. I later realized that swaddling had been utilized in newborn nurseries in hospitals throughout the nation after he was published in a pediatric journal. His ideas were first used in a major hospital that had a future Surgeon General on its staff. Dr. Wilcox later wrote a classic little book about achieving composure or equanimity very early in life and how a colicky baby presents more of a challenge for parents than a placid baby. But the sooner the baby is able to calm down, the better his or her future is concerning living a happy, productive adult life. Again, controlling an overreaction to sensory stimuli is the secret.

HOMEOPATHY AND COLIC

There are combination homeopathic remedies specifically for colic on the over-the-counter market. I (AWS) know a number of parents who have reported good results with these. The most important single remedy is chamomile (*Chamomilla,* abbreviated Cham). This may also be administered as a tea, after being cooled to body temperature. Other herbal ideas are dill, fennel, or caraway. Steep one teaspoon in one cup boiling water. When it cools, give the baby little sips from a spoon, or a little in a bottle. It doesn't take much to help.

Swaddling is most effective as a preventive technique, but it can also ease a full-blown crying episode. Colicky times usually follow a pattern, so swaddling can be employed preceding the feeding that is often followed with a spell of colic. Being relaxed during a feeding (breast or bottle) obviates gulping air—the real culprit, coupled with tenseness. The usual post-feeding burping will be successful when the baby is relaxed. If it is obvious that he is content, he can be put down, still swaddled, on his side. If a bit squirmy, use a portable infant car seat. Certainly, swaddling will not be used except when anticipating or relieving real fussy times. Colic pretty well drops out of the picture after three months. Even during this time, swaddling should not be used continuously but only to control fussy periods.

We will deal further with sleeping position as part of the discussion on sudden infant death syndrome (SIDS). I have always advised putting active babies down on their tummies (the "prone" position), since they seem to seek that more secure position. When swaddled, though, the only acceptable position is the contour-chair position. Currently, a doctor advising putting babies down in the prone position (or even on their side) is considered a heretic in pediatric ranks; so this will need to be discussed with your doctor. When fully informed, I feel sleep position is a parent's choice to make—and that is my position on position.

We have described the cause of most colic and its treatment. There are other causes with different solutions. There is more about food allergy in the feeding chapter. This can be a factor creating great discomfort in the stomach or the intestinal tract. Cow's milk, the base of all but special infant formulas, is a common allergen. In rare cases allergy-producing substances can be transmitted from the mother through her breast milk.

Cramping and a bloody diarrhea signal that something is radically wrong and requires a definitive diagnosis and treatment. The good news is that the problem can be completely overcome by correcting the cause. Intestinal infections, both viral and bacterial, can produce temporary cramping and pain. Inappropriate feeding of foods that are too coarse or that are offered too soon in life can produce a mechanical irritation of the bowel and cause cramping or even mucus in the stools. These more rare causes of colic should be considered if it is not responding to the suggestions of this chapter.

DIARRHEA IN INFANTS AND TODDLERS

Now we must deal with an obnoxious subject but a common one—
so let's get started. The most common form of diarrhea is associated
with a virus infection that begins with vomiting. Rotavirus is the
best-known virus, because it is a worldwide pathogen and because
a vaccine has been developed to reduce the incidence of this easily
spread disease. The first version of the vaccine was associated with
the serious side effect of intussusception, thus creating notoriety.
(See "The Floodgates Open" section in the Immunizations chapter
for more details.)

But there are numerous other viral and bacterial agents that can
infect and cause these symptoms. Norwalk virus, of cruise-ship
fame, has a very short incubation period and spreads like wildfire.
("Norwalk" virus has had a name change to "norovirus." It seems
that the townsfolk of Norwalk, Ohio, where the virus was isolated
and named, no longer wish to be associated with such an obnoxious
infectious agent.)

A small child or infant has little reserve and readily gets into trouble from dehydration and electrolyte (blood salts) loss if the double
whammy of vomiting *and* diarrhea cannot be stopped. I dreaded epidemics of this sort, not just because vomiting and diarrhea are very
messy, but because these illnesses can be unpredictably stubborn.

Vomiting in Infectious Diarrhea

At least vomiting paints a clear picture that something is wrong and
that corrective measures should be started immediately. These illnesses
are very infectious and spread hand to mouth, so another family member who is experiencing similar signs and symptoms could sound the
alarm. Older children and adults with one of these infections often feel
nauseated but might not get to the point of actually vomiting before
diarrhea begins. The older patient, who can describe what is going on,
often complains of cramping and distension (bellyache)—a feeling that
getting things "moving" would provide relief. And it does. The worst
misery is during the pre-diarrhea phase and is relieved as soon as diarrhea begins.

Vomiting can be very difficult to control. It may stubbornly continue even though nothing comes up from retching other than the mucus secreted by the stomach lining. Obviously, regular feedings are out of the question in this situation. Lightly sugared drinks (no artificial "sugars"), usually considered unhealthy, are useful at this time. At first, only sips of plain water will stay down. An infant or toddler may be started on a caffeine-free soft drink such as ginger ale, 7-Up, or Sprite. For infants, a little "defizzing" by stirring is in order. Progress to larger amounts—one ounce for infants and two ounces for toddlers. If only small amounts can be tolerated they must be offered very frequently, even spoon-fed, in an attempt to avoid dehydration. A "good" diet has to be abandoned in favor of getting *some* energy-building calories to stay down, along with water and a little salt. Once larger volumes of liquids are successfully retained, refined starches, such as rice baby cereal and soda crackers can be started. As with the liquids, begin with small amounts offered frequently, and progress by increasing the amounts and interval between feedings. Most fruits and vegetables and meat should be avoided, but normally ripe banana (or banana flakes) is useful in that it encourages the proliferation of "good" bacteria in the gut and is easily digested.

When the child is well past vomiting clear liquids and bits of starchy foods, begin offerings of cultured yogurt, which is of great benefit for shortening the severity and the length of time of diarrhea. Even infants allergic to cow's milk can tolerate yogurt (see the allergy chapter). If the infant or toddler seems prone to developing these infections with some frequency, consider providing a daily intake of beneficial bacteria once they are well. This has been shown to have a preventive function.

Breast-feeding can proceed as soon as vomiting is over. Don't worry about schedule—just nurse when the little one is hungry. If the baby is bottle-fed, this milk contains fat that normally delays stomach emptying, so start with small feedings of two ounces no oftener than at two hour intervals. If your little one has graduated from formula to regular milk, offer "low fat," but not "no fat" milk. Then increase the volume and interval between feedings. Follow the mantra of "proceed cautiously" in getting back to normal. Back off if there is a flare-up of diarrhea, and back off further if vomiting recurs.

The Stools in Infectious Diarrhea

The stools (that strange medical word for bowel movements) produced from a viral, common form of diarrhea may vary in color, depending on its severity. They may be green if they are zipping through the intestinal tract too fast for the bilirubin to oxidize to its normal yellow-brown color. At first, they may be all liquid. They never have the normal baby, buttermilk odor; instead they have a "sick" odor. There may be some mucus. Heavy mucus with flecks of blood, usually accompanied by intestinal cramping, indicates the need for medical examination to check for the possibility of a bacterial diarrhea that requires treatment—the sooner the better. If you feel comfortable with your doctor, just report to his or her office.

The list of pathogens, viral or bacterial, causing these outbreaks of diarrhea is long. Doctors in touch with their local Public Health Office can be alerted about pathogens that are causing trouble in their community, thus narrowing down the suspects, some of which might be potent pathogens.

Hydration

It is very important to keep the infant or toddler hydrated during a bout of infectious diarrhea. Judge hydration by the number of wet diapers and how dark the urine is in them. Sunken eyes and dry lips point to more severe dehydration. There often is electrolyte loss with continuing vomiting and diarrhea. Medical professionals evaluate this by assessing skin turgor. Normally, when the skin over the abdomen is pulled up and then let go, it quickly goes back to its original position. When there is more severe dehydration with electrolyte loss, it goes back slowly. A doctor visit is needed if the child is in this stage of dehydration. Ironically, vomiting and diarrhea worsen with electrolyte loss, accelerating the downhill course. The condition responds dramatically to intravenous fluids, which stop the cycle. Over-the-counter balanced electrolyte solutions can be started at the first hints of dehydration. Once the infant or toddler is stabilized it will be possible to go back to the gradual feeding regimen described above.

CHAPTER 5

FEEDING THE INFANT AND TODDLER AND RELATED PROBLEMS

The feeding of infants has a strong instinctive basis. A characteristic of mammals, humans included, is that they suckle their young; all female mammalians have built-in milk producers and suppliers—their mammary glands.

Infants are nursed at the breast in poor countries because there is no alternative. Well, almost no alternative. In the 1970s, Nestle Company was supplying its infant formula to hospitals and clinics in third world countries. It attempted to promote bottle-feeding as a more "modern" way to nourish infants. The formula was free for new mothers while they were confined and on the day of discharge from the birthing facility. From then on, it was no longer free. A boycott was organized in 1977 to put a stop to this practice, which was not feasible for many reasons.

A common public health problem throughout the undeveloped world is the lack of availability of potable water. Refrigeration of a liquid formula, or any type of milk, is out of the question. The Nestle solution was to make a powdered formula that can be mixed with water at the proper concentration, but mothers were on their own to figure out how they would find safe water. In some areas, it is even difficult to find fuel for making water safe by boiling. It was nearly impossible to overthrow an almost inborn knowledge of infant feeding, developed over eons, for this "modern" method. And to make their purchases last longer, some mothers were mixing the powder with more water than recommended, literally starving their babies. Clearly, this "modern" intervention was not an improvement.

THE PHYSIOLOGY OF BREAST-FEEDING

As soon as the newborn is brought to the breast and "latches on," marvelous interactions of the physical and the nearly spiritual, positive feelings come into play. This is brought about through the area of the brain where emotions (good feelings) and experiences stimulate the pituitary gland to release hormones. One of these, oxytocin, causes contractions of the uterus, shutting down uterine bleeding after the placenta separates and is "born." Another, prolactin, stimulates oxytocin to create milk "let-down" through the sensory aspects of nursing. This allows filling of the ducts surrounding the nipple.

This interplay between the feelings and the mechanics of nursing provides a large contribution to the bonding between mother and infant. Nursing goes a lot more smoothly when these natural factors are allowed to function. When a mother has the feeling that she is successfully providing her infant with more than just a feeding, the interconnection of good feelings and hormone release enhance the process. When "let-down" is consistent, she knows she has arrived. Birthing specialists interested in helping a new mother enjoy success in nursing have found that it is best to put the infant to the mother's breast as soon as possible after delivery. This is the time when the infant, reflexively, gets a better hold on the breast in a manner that will more effectively "milk" the filled ducts that surround the nipple. And the sooner the better for kicking in the oxytocin effect.

Nursing is well known, in both animal husbandry and in humans, as a birth control method that delays the restart of menses. This is another example of breast stimulation and hormone release—not as reliable as the pill, but useful, especially in third world cultures. Unlike hormonal birth control, nursing creates no possibility of undesirable side effects. On the other hand, many a mother has nursed and still had another baby come along unexpectedly soon. Useful does not mean reliable. Nurse for the health of your child, not for family planning.

WHY BREAST-FEEDING IS SUPERIOR

There are so many "perks" to breast-feeding. Let us describe a few. Breast milk passes on maternal antibodies to many infectious diseases. Colostrum, the very first milk after birth, is especially rich in antibodies and other proteins. The antibodies of colostrum are resistant to an enzyme (trypsin), contained in gastric juices, that would otherwise digest the antibodies (and proteins in general). Thus, antibodies against bacterial intestinal pathogens are preserved. In developed countries, viral pathogens that cause diarrhea illnesses predominate. In underdeveloped parts of the world, bacterial pathogens predominate. This is a very strong argument for nursing in areas where babies are subject to die from waterborne infections like diarrhea. Colostrum also works like a laxative to break up the sticky content of the newborn's intestinal tract, called meconium. As soon as a baby is born and is no longer dependent on its mother's circulation for oxygen and nutrients, his or her blood volume is reduced. The resultant breakdown of red blood cells produces bilirubin, which becomes inspissated (thickened) in the meconium. So breast milk plays an important role in ridding the intestinal tract of meconium, which helps make way for the establishment of a healthy bacterial flora.

Superiority of Breast Milk

Some experts unabashedly state: "Breast-feeding is the healthiest form of milk for humans."[1] Before milk formulas were available, early in the twentieth century, mothers nursed their infants, often for two years or more. If she couldn't nurse because of maternal illness, or simply that she chose not to for a variety of reasons, a "wet nurse" came to the rescue. In the South around the time of the Civil War the duty was performed by a slave . . . a new mother, or one who was ready to wean her own. Many times, long after the child was weaned, the wet nurse took on the different role of surrogate mother or nurse. The "wet nurse" was well accepted throughout history, since this was the only way a newborn could survive. This attitude changed with the advent of infant feeding formulas. Today there are breast milk "banks," designed for collecting and distributing breast milk for special-needs hospitalized babies who are unable to use these commercial products.

Unlike formula, breast milk requires no preparation and is always at the proper temperature. It encourages the establishment of the good intestinal flora, *Lactobacillus bifidus*, through the action of a breast-milk growth factor.

Planning Ahead

The question of whether or not to nurse should be asked as soon as a prospective mother begins prenatal care. Education should have no hint of coercion. There may be medical reasons for prohibiting nursing in some cases. Formula feeding has drawbacks when compared to breast-feeding, but infants *can* thrive with formula feeding when breast-feeding cannot be entertained. Recognition of this will help ease the feeling that one might not be a first-class mother if she doesn't nurse.

If nursing is awarded an "A," new formulas should get at least a "B." Nearly all the good things of nursing can be duplicated—if not quite as perfectly—with bottle-feeding. However, except in a case of a definite "no" to breast-feeding, a decision should not be made until all fears of the unknown have been cleared away and possibilities of overcoming foreseen obstacles are discussed. Many offices of doctors in a baby delivering practice, hospitals, and birthing centers have staff members who give expert advice concerning nursing. Being prepared ahead of time makes it all so much easier. A solid start, within minutes of delivery, simplifies the whole process. Unfortunately, an August 3, 2011, message from the Centers for Disease Control reported that a survey of hospitals in the United States found miserable compliance (only 14 percent of hospitals) in their utilization of the World Health Organization (WHO) breast-feeding education and help protocol.

Working moms will need to choose between bottle-feeding or breast-feeding. Even a short maternity leave can get the ball rolling. There are workplaces that accommodate a nursing employee with nursing breaks rather than coffee breaks. This is ideal. It is more cumbersome, and many advantages are lost, but a mother can collect breast milk in baby bottles and refrigerate it for use by another care-taker. A nursing expert can teach the safe methods of collecting breast milk for bottle-feeding. The biggest drawback of supplemental bottle-feeding of either breast milk or formula is that it can easily reduce breast milk production. To achieve optimal production, the breast has to be emptied fairly frequently.

Consider this in making a choice: For successful feeding by either method, contentment is a must. There is no room for feelings of harassment or frustration.

Burping

Whether breast-feeding or bottle-feeding, it is good to learn the fine art of burping. Infants swallow a certain amount of air during feeding. Since air rises to the top, the infant is placed in the upright position, over the parent's shoulder, and gently patted. (I use the word "parent" here, for this is a great way for a father to be an active participant in the care for his baby.) Patting accompanied by rocking, dancing, singing—whatever is relaxing to parent and infant—doesn't just dislodge the bubble of air, it also allows relaxation of the upper stomach valve. This is often done halfway through a feeding and again at the end. If baby gets fussy a short time after being put down, he or she may need more burping.

Breast-Feeding Difficulties and Tips

There can be bumps in the "nursing road" that are smoothed by simple remedies and helpful advice. Breast-feeding specialists, trained in the methods of the La Leche League, are very helpful. It is most beneficial to have help from the experts for several days (as an outpatient service) in order to firmly establish breast-feeding.

A healthy infant gets about 50 percent of the milk from one breast in the first two minutes; and 80 to 90 percent in four minutes. With this information in mind, mother and specialist can see what works best to ease or prevent breast and nipple soreness: to empty one breast completely at a feeding; or two minutes on one side and complete emptying of the second side, depending on breast fullness at the start of feeding. Alternate the procedure the next feeding. Many new mothers experience sore nipples when they start to nurse their newborns. More than just discomfort, this can lead to cracked nipples and, rarely, even mastitis (infection). One good way to prevent this problem before it has to be treated medically is topical application of vitamin E. Dry the nipple and the surrounding breast gently. With a needle or pushpin, make a hole in each end of a vitamin E capsule and squeeze a few drops out directly from the capsule onto this area. You can rub it in gently, or, if the area is really sore, just let it soak in. A trace of vitamin E that may remain on the nipple for the infant—this is a good thing, a side benefit, not a side effect. Cocoa butter and olive oil are other natural alternatives to the chemical ingredients in conventional creams and lotions.

Infant-Related Feeding Difficulties

If the newborn is not actively sucking on anything available, he or she should be thoroughly evaluated as soon as possible to determine what, of a myriad of things, could be causing this lack of enthusiasm. It is normal for a newborn to be a bit groggy for the first day. Sucking reflex and ease of swallowing should be assessed if there seems to be a problem at this time. Physical examination could reveal a very tangible, physical impediment to nursing, such as the not unusual condition of "tongue tie," which makes it nearly impossible for even a vigorous baby to nurse. With tongue tie, the band of fibrous tissue that is usually about midway on the underside of the tongue, anchoring it to the floor of the mouth, is misplaced forward, close to the tip. There are no nerve endings in this tissue; so no pain is inflicted when it is clipped with scissors. (The trick is in getting the baby to hold still.) Your pediatrician can take care of this in an office visit. Since there are no blood vessels or nerve endings in the frenulum, if the baby is still, it is not much worse than clipping a finger nail.

Mother-Related Feeding Difficulties

Occasionally, a mother's nipples will not protrude at feeding time—a very frustrating situation for both mother and infant. There are ways to help draw out inverted nipples. The simplest is doing nothing: Many inverted nipples actually aren't, and what looks like a potential problem will self-correct in the final weeks of pregnancy as the breast prepares for nursing. Also, babies characteristically grab more than the nipple: They get hold of the surrounding area (areola) as well as the nipple. If the issue does not self-correct, a gentle massage or drawing out the nipple with the fingers often works. And, without putting too fine a point on it, so can the loving mouth of an amorous father. Breast shells and nipple shields may be discussed with your birthing specialist if the above methods don't do the trick. But do not dismiss the low-tech ways without trying them.

Sore nipples caused by cracking can be prevented by down-to-business feedings that limit the time on the breast, and with proper cleansing and drying. Mastitis, or breast infection, most often gets underway from stopped-up ducts in the breast(s). It is important to empty the breast at least with every other feeding. It's important, so we want to say it again: One of the best ways to prevent sore and/or cracked nipples is vitamin E. Topical application of vitamin E, right from the capsule as described above, is easy, sanitary, and feels good. (Remember, the nipple and surrounding area needs to be dried first.) If too sore, consider using a nipple shield to bypass the sore nipple until some healing takes place. Mothers who take supplemental vitamin C supplements are less likely to develop mastitis. Vitamin C boosts the immune system, reduces inflammation, and helps fight infection. Frederick R. Klenner, M.D., had all pregnant women in his care take several thousand milligrams of vitamin C per day throughout their pregnancy, and more in the third trimester. We discuss vitamin C in its own chapter, later in this book.

There is no more effective way to reduce milk production than worry. Not that worry *ever* has a place in the scheme of things, but worrying in the first few days about the infant's caloric intake is unproductive, to say the least. Apparently, adjusting to the world on the outside takes a few days, but then the infant will begin to feed in a more predictable manner.

A NUTRITIONAL COMPARISON OF COW'S MILK AND BREAST MILK

Early cow's milk formulas were made of evaporated milk, which started out sterilized. Using breast milk as the benchmark, the two were compared and products rapidly developed that came as close as limited knowledge permitted. Trying to duplicate breast milk required different carbohydrate and protein sources that would make the percentages comparable, while making some sacrifices of quality. Some vitamins were added to close the gap. Calories per ounce were similar . . . about twenty calories per ounce. Although formulas have improved, the two still differ widely in protein content and type. The biggest problem with designing a formula is that, at best, you can only put in it what you already know is in breast milk. In the 1940s and 1950s, vitamins such as vitamin E and biotin were not even regarded as necessary additions.

Progress in Baby Formulas

Going from evaporated milk formulas to the more sophisticated formulas available today met with some bumps in the road along the way. When formulas were first introduced in the 1950s, children's hospitals started admitting infants with seizures who were being fed with one of the new formulas. Tests to rule in or out common causes of seizures were all negative. Some observers brilliantly made the connection that the seizures were possibly related to pyridoxine (vitamin B_6) deficiency, and this detective work proved to be life saving for infants then and in the future. The manufacturer promptly fixed the problem with its product. Pyridoxine is heat labile (altered by heat), and the original product had undergone a heat sterilization process without adding back the destroyed B_6. The proof of the diagnosis was made when the seizures immediately stopped after the affected infant was administered intravenous pyridoxine, at a dosage level many times that of the recommended dietary allowance (RDA) for an adult. Once the deficiency was corrected, the low levels of B_6 obtained from ordinary feeding kept the infant seizure free.

There have been many changes in the composition of the fats in formulas since the rapid increase in knowledge about the various fats: saturated fats, cholesterol, polyunsaturated fatty acids (both omega-3s and omega-6s), and monounsaturated fatty acids. Market forces are influenced by whichever fat is currently under medical fire or is being touted by the medical profession. A look in the grocery store at the formula section will show general agreement among the different brands in the composition of added fats to simulate breast milk.

It's important to keep in mind, however, that a formula of fixed composition is not going to accomplish what breast milk can. Breast milk composition seemingly automatically adjusts to the needs of a rapidly growing infant. Initially, cholesterol content is quite high in breast milk, but these levels lower later. With all the talk of "bad" cholesterol, a formula for a newborn would never sell if the buyer was aware that this "dangerous" substance had been added in order to approximate the level found in breast milk.

Baby Formulas—"Improving" on Nature

What Michael Pollan, well-known writer and food activist, refers to as "nutritionism" is in full force as it applies to the development of formulas suitable for nourishing infants. By this term, Mr. Pollan is referring to the practice of isolating some good components of foods and rearranging them to form a food equal to, or better than, nature's—or so the thinking goes.

When it comes to infant nutrition, human milk should be the ideal, the benchmark. If a supposed "deficiency" is found in it, there should be a lot of thought given before adding the substance in question to a standard baby formula. Samuel J. Foman, M.D., Professor of Pediatrics at the University of Iowa College of Medicine and author of *Infant Nutrition,* was considered to be the authority on infant nutrition. He and many other authorities feel that human milk is deficient in vitamin D and fluoride. (While at the same time, they warn of fluoride toxicity.) Yet there is no clinical evidence of these deficiencies unless the mother herself suffers from them. It seems that sun exposure is the main source of vitamin D for humans, and that the smaller amount in the breast milk from a healthy mother with adequate vitamin D in her bloodstream will be adequate for the baby. Dark-skinned mothers who do not produce adequate vitamin D from sunlight, or mothers kept from sunshine by clothing or sunscreen protection definitely need vitamin D supplementation. Fluoride is a *trace* mineral and, along with other trace minerals, was not even considered in breast milk composition tables until fluoridation of water supplies became an issue.[2] What works best for calves and human babies are two different things.

Proteins, Carbohydrates, and Other Nutritional Elements

Cow's milk has twice the protein content, and its protein consists of nearly seven times more casein, than human milk. This means that human milk has more whey protein and less of the more allergenic casein. These factors favor the formation of a smaller, more digestible curd in the digestive system and provide an intestinal pH that supports colonization with *Lactobacillus bifidus* (a probiotic) in the breast-fed baby.

The carbohydrate lactose, makes up 7 percent of human milk and 4.8 percent of cow's milk. In early evaporated-milk formulas, the carbohydrate difference was made up with dextromaltose (a complex sugar) or corn syrup. More current formulas equalize the carbohydrate content with more lactose or, still, even corn syrup (fructose). The total fat content is equal, but in human milk, polyunsaturated fatty acids make up 8 percent of the total, while in cow's milk it is only 2 percent of the total.

Docosahexaenoic acid (DHA) the long-chain omega-3 fatty acid, naturally derived from the fat of cold-water fish, has gained much acclaim the last few years. (Some DHA can be synthesized in the body from other fatty acids, but fish oils contain a high concentration.) It and eicosapentaenoic acid (EPA) are known to be precursors of the anti-inflammatory prostaglandins. Since inflammation is a part of so many disorders, these fatty acids have received a lot of attention. DHA has also been found to have a prominent role in brain and retina development. By weight, 60 percent of the brain consists of fats. (Note: This still does not justify calling someone a fathead.) DHA makes up 40 percent of the fats in the brain and 60 percent in the retina. Maternal dietary intake has been shown to nourish the developing brain and retina in both the fetus and the newborn. Breast milk content varies with the mother's intake, while some formulas don't contain any at all.

If the mother's intake of omega-6 fatty acid is elevated, omega-3 fatty acids are reduced in her milk. A teeter-totter-like balance rules. (The omega-6 fatty acid, although required by the human body, is a precursor to *pro*inflammatory prostaglandins and considered to be a factor in the development of many diseases.) A study on the changes in the consumption of omega-3 and omega-6 in the United States found that between 1945 and 1995, linoleic acid (the omega-6 essential fatty acid) made up 6 to 7 percent of the total fat of breast milk. This figure went from 6 percent in the 1960s to 18 percent in 1986. The authors felt this was due to a great increase in the use of soybean oil as well as more grain fed than pasture raised animals.[3] There are many studies showing tangible evidence of the benefits of DHA for both vision and intelligence. I noticed one formula in particular that boasted having added DHA to its contents, and it may be included in others. One author, in the online article *Breast Milk Can Not Be Imitated—The DHA/ARA Fallout and Oligosaccharides,* writes that the DHA that is added to formulas is synthesized, is known to produce side effects, and doesn't come close to resembling the natural DHA of breast milk.[4]

An oligosaccharide is a sugarlike molecule consisting of a short chain of several simple sugars linked together. They make up the third

THE MEANING OF "ESSENTIAL"

Most get the picture of the word root of vitamins—vital for health. Many more understand that our bodies do not manufacturer these vital substances. We have to get them from our diet or as nutrition supplements. I am amazed at the number of those who have no idea of the meaning of essential fatty acids. What is there about the word "essential" that they don't understand? My thought is that even intelligent, informed (but incorrectly informed) people have been duped by those who would demonize "fat" of any kind.

I had only a single case of severe essential fatty acid deficiency in an infant. The baby was about nine months old. Length was compatible with this age, but weight was below the fifth percentile. The baby's skin was dry and lusterless. There was muscle wasting with flat buttocks, dry mouth and lips. In short, he looked like a victim of famine.

When I began my taking a dietary history, it got very interesting. His mother was a staunch believer in the evils of fat and had put the infant on skim milk several months ago. It was a situation that had to be remedied as quickly as possible. I was aware that I had to be careful about the way I approached the problem so that I wouldn't be the cause of too much guilt. However, I wasn't able to produce any guilt feelings. She didn't buy my advice and promptly told me so. She could not understand that I, supposedly an intelligent doctor, didn't go along with all the other doctors who condemned fat. She snatched up the infant and left. I have often wondered what happened to the little one. I pray that, somehow, facing the facts would come through. Or perhaps some of the mother's friends might ask why the baby was so scrawny.

largest solid component of breast milk, following lactose and lipids. Overall, they aid the establishment of a favorable intestinal flora. Special-use formulas have been developed for numerous common infant problems by manipulating these individual ingredients and by considering the actions of specific amino acids (the building blocks of proteins). Thus, there are special formulas for differing growth stages and for specific conditions: being born prematurely, restless sleep, excess gas, immune system support, tendency to develop milk allergy, or having milk allergy. One label states that the formula was designed for "colic" (printed in big letters). Below this, in very tiny letters: "due to protein sensitivity." This product consists of hydrolyzed milk proteins, especially the more allergy-prone casein. This same product was used almost exclusively for severe cow's milk sensitivity—*50 years ago.* Hydrolyzation is a process that breaks proteins down into their amino acid building blocks, rendering the protein unable to provoke an allergic reaction. (What amazed me about this product was the way infants who needed this formula would lap it up, even though it smelled and tasted much like library paste.) The "immune system support" formula comes closest to the breast-milk ratio of the two milk proteins, casein and whey (the latter being the less allergenic).

With all this scientific tweaking, formulas are still runners-up to breast milk. But they are a good second choice when breast-feeding can't be considered. Babies thrived with less sophisticated evaporated milk formulas in the past, and they can with these. They also open the window for someone other than the mother to feed and show love to her baby when she is not able to nurse.

Vitamins and Minerals in Formulas and Breast Milk

The vitamin content of several current brand-name infant feeding formulas is similar. In general, the labels list the content in portions of 100 calories per five ounces. Assuming six feedings in twenty-four hours at five ounces per feeding, an infant would consume about one liter (which is what most composition tables are based on). Of course, the size of the feeding must be an average over the entire first year of life.

The fat-soluble vitamins, with the exception of vitamin K, show human milk superiority. Except for vitamin C, the other water-soluble vitamins such as the Bs are in much greater concentration in cow's milk. This leads to my speculation that the content of both the bovine and the human mothers' milk is influenced by what she eats and what her offspring needs. I am certain that if human mothers had the digestive tract of a cow and grazed on lush grass all day long, or if the mother cow didn't have to supply her calf with B vitamins and vitamin K until it could graze, there might be equality in the vitamin content of their milk. Not only that, cows and calves make their own vitamin C. So do mares and their foals. So do bears and their cubs, geese and their goslings, dogs and their puppies, cats and their kittens, frogs with their tadpoles, and even insects and their buglets. (Disclaimer: "buglet" is not a real term.) In fact, practically every animal in creation makes their own vitamin C. Humans cannot. Neither can the apes, monkeys, fruit bats, or guinea pigs. We need extra vitamin C, and we will go into this in detail in the Vitamin C chapter later in this book.

Vitamin A

Doing the calculations for vitamin A, 300 International Units (IU) per five ounces comes close to providing the 1,500 IU per day that is based on the recommended dietary allowance (RDA). Many consider this to be way too low a standard. (We will get to that later, when vitamin supplements are discussed.) The RDA for vitamin A varies from 1,320 IUs for the first six months to 1,650 IUs the next six months. The safest way to get more vitamin A into your weaned baby or toddler is to feed carotene-rich orange vegetables. This is, to mix a metaphor, a piece of cake. Kids love sweet potatoes and pumpkin pie, and you will be surprised how many children enjoy winter squash served with butter and a judicious dash of salt. Offer these foods and prepare to be pleased with the results.

Vitamin D

Using the same calculations as for vitamin A, about 300 IUs of vitamin D are present in a quart of formula. There is over one-third more vitamin D in breast milk than in cow's milk.

At last, the inadequacy of the past RDA recommendations for vitamin D, based on staying clear of any possibility of toxicity, is yielding to basing the need on blood levels that will accomplish a desired effect. Like the recommendations for daily vitamin D_3 intake, these figures are continually going up, from 25 nanograms per milliliter (ng/ml) just a few months ago to between 40–60 ng/ml for both children and adults. Dr. Holick (and we strongly agree) feels that deficiency is common in all age groups, so essentially all are at risk. Holick's research reveals that infants need a minimum of 400 IU per day and young children a minimum of 600 IU per day. These are minimum amounts. Upper limits to avoid toxicity are: 1,000 IU for up to six months of age, 1,500 IU for six months to one year of age, 3,000 IU up to eight years of age, and 4,000 IU above eight years. With such a large spread between efficiency and toxicity, increases could be made for conditions that might reduce fat absorption, and also for obesity, a condition which requires two to three times more vitamin D.[5]

Vitamin K

There is four times the level of the other fat-soluble vitamin, vitamin K, in cow's milk than in human milk, probably due to the increased bone metabolism required by the rapidly growing calf and because the mother cow has a good supply in her milk from eating her greens and having a good supply of beneficial, vitamin K-generating bacteria in her digestive system.

Other Vitamins

The water-soluble vitamins, the Bs and vitamin C, are added in minimal amounts to formulas, with those receiving more publicity getting a better shake. And so, down the list of all the vitamins, attempts at coming close to the standard of breast milk are made. Vitamin C, which is destroyed by heat, is even lost when it is dissolved in liquid. Parents using formula can fortify it with extra vitamin C. The non-acidic form, calcium ascorbate, is the one to use for this purpose. A quarter of a teaspoon of calcium ascorbate contains 1,000 mg of vitamin C. This means that you do not have to add more than a smidgen. For those not familiar with smidgens, it is smaller than a skosh and larger than a trace. (Kidding a bit.) The amount of vitamin C to use for formula-fed infants is about 50 mg per feeding, which is a twentieth of a quarter-teaspoon. Breast-feeding mothers can simply increase their own supplemental vitamin C intake to increase the vitamin C in their breast milk. For a nursing mom, 3,000 to 6,000 mg per day, divided up into all-through-the-day 1,000 mg doses, would be what Dr. Klenner and other orthomolecular physicians would suggest.

Minerals

Attention should also be paid to the mineral content of cow's milk versus breast milk. Cow's milk has over three times the concentration of calcium, over six times as much phosphorus, and three times the magnesium of human milk. Sodium, chloride, and potassium concentrations are also around three times higher. I believe we can account for this disparity by considering the differences in maturity at birth and growth rates of calves and human infants. The newborn calf is on its feet (hooves) and beginning its accelerated growth during its first day of life. This difference alone shows why there is a much greater need in cow's milk for the minerals that build bone. This same need does not exist in the human infant, who grows at a much slower pace and therefore has different requirements for these minerals.

There is good equality between human and cow's milk in trace minerals, even in iron. The irony of iron is that subtle microbleeding in the intestinal tract of infants often accompanies cow's milk ingestion. This can lead to anemia; so there is a need for iron fortification to correct iron-deficiency anemia. The formula formulators are very careful not to put what they consider too much of anything in. So safety is assured.

VITAMIN SUPPLEMENTS

Since the most-prescribed (suggested) infant vitamins are produced by the same companies that make infant formulas, it is not surprising to find the same minimal doses in both the formulas and the vitamin drops. Rather than attempting to provide a product with optimal amounts of vitamins and minerals, manufacturers are obsessed with staying within the "safe" range provided by the RDAs set by the U.S. Food and Drug Administration (FDA). These recommendations are set to provide the minimum amount that will prevent an associated deficiency disease, such as rickets from vitamin D deficiency, or beriberi from thiamin (B_1) deficiency—very safe in terms of having no possibility of providing a toxic dose. Their concept of what constitutes a toxic amount of a supplement is unsupported by clinical studies, however. Current vitamin D recommendations are a good example of this problem: The "experts" have been all over the map when it comes to recommended dosage. The recommended dosage for infants, according to the American Academy of Pediatrics in 1998, was only 200 IUs per day, with claims of exceeding safety standards if more were given. Present research seems to find no level that exceeds safety levels. Whatever happened to vitamin D toxicity?

The makers of infant formulas feel so confident about the adequacy of the vitamin content of their formulas that the vitamin-drop supplements of similar composition are suggested only for breast-fed infants. Isn't that an interesting twist? Formula is adequate. Nature's own formula doesn't fill the bill.

For the accessible vitamin preparations, available in supermarkets or drug stores, these puny formulations prevail. There is no evidence

VITAMIN E

In addition to a good no-junk-food diet, daily multivitamins, and vitamin C supplements, vitamin E is easy to give to very young children. A drop or two can be squeezed into their mouth. *My* (AWS) kids liked it, even as infants. Yours may or may not. If they do not, try a chewable dry (succinate) form of vitamin E. Only a small fraction of a tablet will do the trick, and the trick is to give *at least* the too-low U.S. RDA. The vitamin E content of foods is very low. It is literally impossible to design a diet a child will actually eat that provides enough. Supplementing with this valuable antioxidant is also very safe.

Overexposure to oxygen has been a major cause of retrolental fibroplasia (retinopathy of prematurity) and subsequent blindness in premature infants. Incubator oxygen retina damage is now prevented by giving preemies 100 milligrams (mg) of vitamin E per kilogram of body weight. That dose is equivalent to an adult dose of over 5,000 IU for an average weight adult. "There have been no detrimental side effects" from such treatment, according to the *New England Journal of Medicine*.[1] Nevertheless, the sixth edition of the textbook *Nutrition and Diet Therapy* advised that "healthy persons stand the chance of developing signs of toxicity with the megadoses that are recommended in these studies."[2] That incorrect statement was dropped in the book's next edition. Instead, the seventh edition said under "Toxicity Effects" that "Vitamin E is the only one of the fat-soluble vitamins for which no toxic effect in humans is known. Its use as a supplement has not shown harmful effects."[3]

References

1. Hittner, H. M., L. B. Godio, A. J. Rudolph, et al. "Retrolental Fibroplasia: Efficacy of Vitamin E in a Double-Blind Clinical Study of Preterm Infants." *N Engl J Med* 305(23) (Dec 3, 1981):1365–1371.

2. Williams, S. R. Nutrition and Diet Therapy, 6th ed., St. Louis: Times Mirror/Mosby, 1989, p225.

3. Williams, S. R. Nutrition and Diet Therapy, 7th ed., St. Louis: Mosby, 1993, p 186.

that they do harm with the exception of those that include fluoride. I recommend finding preparations, perhaps at a health food store, that contain at least 400 IU of vitamin D (the standard fifty years ago) and 3,000 to 5,000 IU of vitamin A (two to three times the amount in the "safe" preparation). The pro-vitamin A substance, beta-carotene, is safe at any amount found in an infant vitamin preparation. The same thing is true for vitamin E—get all you can without fear of too much. For a normally healthy infant, even the puny amounts of the B vitamins are probably all right for the first year of life. Extra B vitamins are needed for several conditions that arise in the second year and on. Certainly, one can not find an infant multivitamin with too much vitamin C; so, in searching for the best preparation, get all the vitamin C you can. In my search for an easy-to-deliver form of a large dose of vitamin C, I started with the trade name Ce-Vi-Sol that was popular among pediatricians many years ago. Regardless of the product you use, for anything like a substantial dose we absolutely have to add more vitamin C to it. Start with the best tasting liquid-vitamin preparation you can find. Yes, try several and see for yourself. If you like it, the baby will, too. Then beef it up by adding one or two thousand mg of extra vitamin C (as calcium ascorbate, mentioned above) to the bottle's contents at least every week. Details on vitamin C will be found in the chapter on high-dose vitamin C therapy.

Multivitamins have been and remain the easiest, safest, and most cost effective way to go orthomolecular (to prevent and treat disease nutritionally). I (AWS) now have dual vantage points: both from a parental and now a grandparental experience. My kids, and now my grandchildren, get vitamin supplements every day. So do I. So should you and your whole family.

Supplements for Babies

Liquid multivitamins for children are easy to obtain and, unless they contain fluoride, are nonprescription. Health food stores or the Internet remain your best shopping choices. Generally, but not always, you get what you pay for. Check the side label of the container, for that's where the details are found. You should be able to see this information whether you are looking at the physical product in a store or are shopping in an online store. Look for products that list more than mere RDA quantities. It is also important what is NOT in the supplement. You may also have to pay more money for less . . . when it comes to supplement additives. Say no to artificial sweeteners, artificial colors, and artificial flavors. We consider a preservative in a liquid vitamin to be reasonable. You do not want it to spoil once it is open. Vote with your dollars: Choose as natural a supplement as you can find and afford.

If money is very tight, you might want to buy any commercial adult liquid vitamin product at a big-box discount store. This low-cost

SO YOU WANT TO BE ON TV?
AND YOU ARE A HEALTH NUT?

It is a rare event when and if a television station airs anything positive about vitamins or negative about fluoridation. (We'll go into this in detail later in the fluoridation chapter.) If it does, a vocal "health nut" may expect to be edited down to a few seconds of your most "passionate" expression. Dr. Robert Cathcart (http://www.orthomed .com), an M.D. who was a megadose vitamin C expert, told me (AWS) that he'd been frequently interviewed and virtually never aired. Back in the 1980s, PBS' *NOVA* did a fine program on Linus Pauling, including his advocacy of vitamin C. It actually showed him and his wife measuring out "about four grams," to quote Dr. Pauling, and mixing it up to drink it down. I have never, ever, seen this specific program in reruns.

It reminds me of when I was teaching high school: Parents with failing kids (if we saw them at all) did not respond well to truthful, thoughtful comments. A principal advised me to pull out the guidebook and show the student's scores, and politely concentrate on nothing but the numbers. If you do get interviewed on a program, may I submit that you follow this same advice. You might want to list five or ten of the best studies and say, "Do you feel this information is important to your coverage of the story, and to your viewers and their doctors?"

If you are not aired satisfactorily, get on the Internet and post your experience there. We are keen on exposing bias.

option has drawbacks, but is far better than nothing. If the product's quantities of each vitamin are only at RDA levels, you can give more of it. Better yet, give it more often.

Supplements for Toddlers

Chewable multiple vitamins are easiest by far to give to a young child. Almost all of them taste delicious. The tastiest are made with natural flavor, and are the most expensive. The very best have no artificial flavors, artificial colors, or fake sweeteners.

How much to give? *The quick answer is, adjust the dose to your child's weight, and round up.* If the average adult weighed 180 pounds, than an 18-pound infant is one-tenth an adult, and would be given one-tenth of an adult dose. If an adult dose of liquid multivitamin is a tablespoon, then the baby would get one-tenth of a tablespoon.

The better answer is a bit longer. Children need a disproportionally high quantity of daily vitamins compared with adults. In other words, if you scaled a child, metabolism and all, up to that 180-pound adult weight (or if you scaled an adult down to a child's weight), you'd find that the *kids need proportionally more nutrition per pound than grownups do.* A look at the U.S. RDAs confirms this. For most vitamins, RDAs for babies are about a quarter of the RDA for a fully grown man or woman, even though a baby weighs only about one-tenth as much as an adult. The RDA of vitamin E for a one-year-old baby is a third of that for an adult. It is even more obvious with vitamin C. The Adequate Intake (AI) (used when an RDA cannot be established) for a seven-month infant is 50 mg; the RDA for a grown adult is 90 mg.

We feel this supports our opinion that multivitamin supplements for children are especially important.

The Cost of Children's Vitamins

Is the cost of children's vitamin supplements bugging you? Oh, please. The average baby goes through between 6,000 and 7,000 diapers before completing toilet training. You might just as well have a healthy baby as a dry baby.

Just raising one kid to age eighteen can cost a quarter of a million dollars, according to the U.S. Department of Agriculture.[7] Do it on a health homesteader's budget, like I (AWS) did, and it's still a hundred grand, easy.

By any standard of comparison, you can afford supplements. Adjusted for 2013 dollars, we personally spent about forty cents a day per child on preventive megadoses of vitamins. That's under a hundred and fifty bucks a year per kid. When they were sick, up went the C and out came the vegetable juicer. But, aside from physicals, there were no doctor visits. (I mean *none*: My son and daughter never even met their pediatricians.) No office call fees; no waiting-room scream-a-thons; no co-pays; no medicines, prescription or otherwise. Such savings certainly covered the cost of carrots for juicing and extra vitamin C.

ADDING SOLID FOODS TO THE DIET

Unlike the cow, we are not set up to be able to digest cellulose and other fibers. Undigested fiber in the diet has many attributes for older children and adults, but not for infants. Fiber moderates the rapid absorption of sugars and refined grains, reducing a hyperinsulin response as well as reducing the transit time of passage of food substances through the intestinal tract—a process helpful in avoiding constipation or irritable bowel syndrome. Fiber, especially soluble fiber, has many other good functions, such as providing a good medium for establishing a beneficial intestinal flora (good bacteria). But no matter how finely foods are ground (pureed) they can never be fully digested. An infant's intestinal tract is equipped to handle nothing other than milk.

Infants apparently can thrive with minimal levels of vitamin and mineral intake, but we can search for more optimal nutrition when they are old enough to be enlarging their diet to include solid foods. The advice regarding when to introduce juices and solid food to infants has been somewhat cyclic, varying between three and six months. Various factors enter into the decision making: Is there a family history of allergy? Are the new foods what the baby wants or what the parents want? Consider the pros and cons of individual foods. The fast-food industry quickly caught on to the fact that sugar and salt make foods appealing. Most of what we consider taste is actually "smell." The basic tastes are salt, sweet, sour, and bitter. Blindfold a person, put a clothespin on his nose, and have him take a bite out of a peach and then an onion: he won't be able to tell the difference.

Babies like the sweetness of breast milk that is provided by lactose, so the thinking went that they would probably like sweet foods and juices for the initial offering of regular foods. The early baby-foods makers, considering this "sweet tooth" of the toothless infant, advised starting solid feedings with pureed fruits and baby cereals. Later, the salt desire was satisfied with pureed vegetables and meat. The commercial baby foods did a decent job of providing convenience and appeal, but they also contained some less-than-desirable ingredients. Even though the texture, much like a thick liquid, did not appeal to adults, I never heard a baby complain. (Although they may have tried!)

All but the baby cereals could then, and can now, be readily duplicated at home, but they must be presented as very finely ground or chopped. Special baby-food food-grinders or blenders are available; some are hand-operated, easily cleanable, and inexpensive. Foods should be *introduced* to the infant and never insisted on. If forced, there will be trouble ahead with the toddler who can't be made to swallow but has learned to throw things in protest. Slipping into the dietary patterns of an older child will come in degrees. Remember, little ones in the third world countries thrive on exclusive breast-feeding for much longer, usually for well over two years of age.

A wonderful change in baby foods has started, which I believe is due to more awareness of the need to steer clear of any additives (or

FORGOTTEN GRAINS

Wheat and corn allergies or sensitivities, which are fairly common, can put the pressure on parents, as such situations limit your grain options. Rice, once popular for its easy digestibility, has recently been called into question due to its botanic ability to take up arsenic from contaminated farm soils. Until we clean our soils well enough so "organic" can truly apply to rice, we need to be mindful of our alternatives.

Good news: There are other grains readily available, at low cost, and organically grown. Oats and barley are excellent, wholesome, complex carbohydrates. Both can be rolled or chopped when dry, prior to packaging. You can also grind up or blend after cooking. I (AWS) had a little white plastic, hand-held mini food mill that I kept at the table for just such a purpose. Thorough cooking with adequate water goes a long way to making even that step optional.

Rolled oats cook quickly, and chopped rolled oats (quick oats) even more quickly. Select "quick" oats, not "instant." Instant oatmeal is typically loaded with salt. That's not what you want for youngsters. Quick oats are just chopped-up, whole rolled oats, and are just as good. The "quick oat" advantages are faster cooking and a creamier, more little-child friendly food.

Barley can be purchased as "pearled" or "whole." The "whole" has more fiber and nutrients than pearled. Both, if completely cooked, are fine, but pearled may be more infant friendly. If you have barely any basis for boiling a better batch of baby barley, please take note: Barley has to be cooked for quite a long while. Barley is whole, and, like steel-cut oats, takes far longer, as both have less surface area.

My first time at bat, I was quite surprised to see how much cooking water it takes to make a soft, baby-palatable product. Follow label cooking directions and when in doubt, use extra water. After it cools, run the cooked barley (or oats, or anything else you choose) through the food mill.

Introduce all foods a tad at a time; every child is different and experience is still the best guide. Do what works. And don't forget potatoes: Sure, they are not grains. But as complex carbos, they fill the bill. No reason (except for oddity) that a toddler can't have mashed potatoes for breakfast. And if you have not tried potato pancakes, you're in for a treat. So are your children!

deviation from the natural when possible) and toxic pesticides. In short, the organic movement is taking hold, and producers of baby foods are on board—possibly largely from consumer pressure. I checked out one "old" baby food company's products. They are vastly improved. Their foods are labeled "first foods" (the fruits and cereals) and "second foods" (the meats and vegetables) for the older infant. All this fits current recommendations of not starting solid foods until six months of age and avoiding the introduction of some of the more common allergy provoking foods. An article in *Archives of Adolescent Medicine* found that delaying introduction of allergenic foods does not provide protection against developing atopic disease[6] (allergic hypersensitivity) after five years of age, but I would be reluctant to completely abandon the concept of postponing introduction of the more common allergens. This company—and I am sure the other major companies are doing the same—has gone above and beyond the call of duty. All of the "first start" foods are *organic and of simple composition*. Wonderful! Apples are organic (that means unsprayed) and have only one other ingredient: vitamin C, a healthful additive. Some of the "first foods" besides vitamin C will also include citric acid (also not a bad additive), choline (a B vitamin), vitamin E, and DHA (the fatty acid important for the developing retinae and brain). Some of the organic vegetables are just "as is" (the vegetable and water), or in the case of sweet potatoes, vitamin C is added to prevent oxidation and color change. Besides "organic" there are brands that are made with 100 percent natural fruits or vegetables, but are not organically grown. (I really can't say what an "unnatural" fruit or vegetable looks like.) There should be little concern about pesticide residue when vegetables are industrially peeled and washed. Fresh, raw fruits (especially grapes) eaten unpeeled and whole really need to be organic, or if not, washed in soap and water (and rinsed, of course) to remove pesticide residues.

The Produce Without the Poison: How to Avoid Pesticides

Cantaloupe: Pop's got the ladder.

(Favorite joke of Mr. Hughes, my [AWS] high school English teacher.)

Real-world people shop at supermarkets, and real-world affordable fruits and vegetables contain pesticide residues. Not everybody can buy organic; not everybody is a gardener. Here are easy and effective ways to reduce your chemical consumption.

Rule number one: Wash your fruits like you wash your hands. "Use soap, Jimmy!" Mom and Dad were right: just running your mitts or your munchies under tap water does little to remove oily grime. Agricultural pesticides do not come off in water, either. If they did, farmers would have to apply them after each rain or even after a heavy dew. That would be both labor intensive and expensive. So petrochemical companies make pesticides with chemical "stickers" that are insoluble in water. They do their job and stay on the fruit, rain or shine.

Soap, or detergent, is more effective in removing pesticide residue than you think. You can prove this for yourself. Take a big bunch of red or green grapes, and place them, with a squirt of dishwashing detergent, in a large bowl or pan of water. Mix the detergent in thoroughly, and swish the grapes around for a minute. Carefully watch the water. You will see evidence that detergent works. If you do not think that the grayish stuff coming off the grapes is pesticide residue, try another bowl of grapes in water without detergent, and try another bowl of organically grown grapes in water with detergent. Seein' is believin'.

It is necessary to rinse detergent-washed fruits before eating, of course, but that is hardly a burden. Rinse until the water is clear. When you handle the detergent-washed fruit, you will also notice that it feels different, too. We are so used to fruit with chemical coatings on it that when we touch truly clean fruit, it's a new tactile experience. Go ahead, try it. Nobody's looking.

Even if you do not believe that pesticides pose the slightest health risk, there is no downside to not eating them. Whatever benefits they may confer on the tree, pesticides do you no good in your gut. Children may consume disproportionally large amounts of pesticides because kids eat a lot of fruit relative to their body weight. For parents, there is a measure of comfort in knowing that their kid's chemical intake has been minimized.

In my opinion, newly detergent-washed fruit does not keep very well. The former petrochemical coating probably served as a moisture barrier and even an oxidation barrier. No worries: You only wash before you eat.

In case you think I am taking too easy-going a view on chemical farming, I would like to point out that I am an avid organic gardener. I also advocate purchasing chemical-free foods whenever possible, including organically grown produce. It costs more to buy organic, but, if you can afford it, it is probably money well spent. Home gardening, on the other hand, is an incredibly cheap alternative. All those stories that you hear about a thirty-dollar investment in seed and fertilizer yielding seven hundred dollars worth of fresh food are literally true. If you think I'm more full of fertilizer than my garden is, I recommend that you try it and see. For starters, you could try leaf lettuce, zucchini squash, cucumbers, bush green beans, and a dozen tomato plants. You will soon be supplying half the neighborhood.

A cheap organic gardening hint: None of the veggies I just mentioned require any pesticides to grow well.

Another cheapskate hint: Save those potatoes that are "no good" because they've sprouted "eyes." Don't throw them away; plant them. The "eyes" are indeed sprouts, each of which will grow into an entire potato plant bearing several, or even many, spuds. Cut the 'tater up and plant each piece with a sprout on it. No pesticides needed here, either.

Pesticides are bug poisons. It is hard to kill an insect. I distinctly recall flea powdering my Basset hound, an activity I performed frequently. I'd dust that dog so well that he looked like one of the Three Stooges with a sack of flour poured on him. There would be heaps of flea powder in the dog's nooks and crannies, and I watched fleas walk and even tunnel through piles of poison powder without ill effect. Bugs are tough little stinkers, all right. And you eat the stuff they try to kill them with. Delish!

So, as it takes a lot of spray to stop a hungry bug, it takes at least a little detergent to remove the spray. Or, you could insist on no sprays, and risk more bugs. Would you buy such produce? No? Then we need to be honest, admit it, and be willing to clean the fruit effectively.

Many fruits and vegetables are not merely sprayed, but are waxed as well. So-called "food grade" waxes improve shelf life and appearance, but coat over and lock in any previously applied pesticides. This poses a problem, because waxes do not readily dissolve in detergent solution. You might find a product or two on the market that is certified to remove waxes from fruits. The other alternative is to simply peel them. Frequently waxed fruits include apples, pears, eggplant, cucumbers, and squash. Even tomatoes are generally waxed. The lack of a high gloss is not proof positive that a fruit is unwaxed: many waxes, like many types of floor polyurethane or spray varnish, are not at all shiny. One way to tell if a fruit or vegetable is waxed is to run your fingernail over it and see if you can scrape anything off. Another way is to read the label and see if the produce is waxed. This may require a trip in back to the warehouse to see the carton that the produce came in. Rotsa' ruck on that.

A peeler costs under a buck, and effectively removes wax. A squirt of dish detergent costs a few cents. The public library costs nothing.

For more pesticide-reducing reading, I recommend:

Center for Science in the Public Interest. *99 Ways to a Simple Lifestyle*. Garden City, NY: Anchor Press, 1977.

Issac, K., S. Gold, ed. *Eating Clean 2: Overcoming Food Hazards.* Washington, D.C.: Center for Study of Responsive Law, 1987.

Kulvinskas, V. *Survival into the 21st Century: Planetary Healers Manual.* Wethersfield, CT: Omangod Press, 1975.

Taub, H. J. *Keeping Healthy in a Polluted World.* NY: Penguin, 1975.

Wigmore, A. *Recipes for Longer Life.* Garden City Park, NY: Avery, 1982.

The Cost of "Organic"

Let's consider the price differential between "organic" and "natural" baby foods. Comparing apples with apples: Five ounces of organic apples are $1.23 in the "first foods" category (24.6 cents per ounce). Organic apples in the "second foods" category are 10.5 percent less expensive than the organic apples in the "first foods" category. Part of the reduction is due to the reduced cost of packaging for the "second foods" product. A cherry-apple combination "Natural Select" product was 22 percent cheaper than the organic "second food" product, and the same product "on sale" was reduced 13 percent further. The "organic" apples in the "first foods" are only 10.6 percent more costly than those in the "second foods" category, but some of the other "first foods," with added DHA, may pass on their added expense to other products in the same group. We do pay for convenience. Even with the extra expense, my thought is to use the "first start" foods for the first few months; then feel comfortable with the "natural" foods, which would contain no pesticide residue, in the "second foods" category. If organic fruits and vegetables are available, "homemade" should do nicely and be less expensive.

Baby cereals are pretty much the same as they have always been. A few everyday foods are recognized as having a high potential for producing food allergies: cow's milk, orange juice, wheat, and eggs. The accepted practice is to delay the introduction of these foods, especially the potent allergen, egg white. With adults sold on the idea that oats are "heart healthy" and that oat bran will take care of cholesterol, it looks like oats, for both reasons, have become the favorite component of baby cereals. Cooked cereal has been the favorite for thickening milk feedings offered to a baby who spits-up too much. These cereals are fine, nutritionally speaking. They have pretty much the additives they have always had: dicalcium and tricalcium phosphates, lecithin, and mixed tocopherols (vitamin E) "to preserve freshness" (actually to prevent rancidity of the grain and the added lecithin). None of this is bad, but it could be duplicated with homemade cereal that is not too coarse and made from the organically grown grain (without additives).

EXTRA WATER AND JUICES

If Mom stays well hydrated, her infant's water needs will be met. Both a breast-fed and a bottle-fed infant might be more satisfied by occasionally offering water from a bottle (sterile, of course) between milk feedings. Hydration is best judged by how wet the diapers are and how often they get that way. More attention needs to be paid to hydration when the ambient temperature is high or during an illness with fever (see the fever chapter). It is a good idea to prepare even the exclusively breast-fed infant to be able to accept a bottle in case of any sort of disruption of nursing.

Juice used to be introduced early. Orange juice was the juice of choice because of its vitamin C and good folic acid content. Then it was noted that the juice was creating allergic reactions in an ever-increasing number of infants and apple juice, with added vitamin C, took its place. Advertising the health value of apple juice created a problem. Pediatricians were seeing infants with distended bellies who were in rather poor shape nutritionwise. Far too much apple juice was displacing formula intake. (This type of trouble, and its solution, makes a real pitch for the "well check.") The problem sneaks up on the parent trying to do the best for her infant, who listens to faulty nutrition advice intended for "bigger" people (adults). It can be easily spotted by a doctor familiar with this common problem.) A little juice is fine, but not essential. Too much creates a "gassy," uncomfortable baby. Whether the juice is made just for infants or off the "general" shelf, check the ingredients label. Regular juices might contain undesirable additions such as high-fructose corn syrup (HFCS), food coloring, and chemical preservatives. The baby juices are not likely to contain these ingredients, which have received so much negative attention. Actually, some might also be organic and have vitamin C as the only thing added to the pure juice.

BPA IN FOOD CONTAINERS

We seem to always be able to find new things to worry about in this toxic environment of ours. One such substance is bisphenol A (BPA), a chemical that is part of many polycarbonate plastics—food-packaging plastics and containers, *and* baby bottles. BPA is released into food by heating, so it seems obvious that this already deemed toxic substance should not be used—especially—for making baby bottles or the containers of baby foods that might be microwave heated.

Many question the FDA standard of toxicity levels for infants, which are notoriously too high for other toxic products. To support the FDA and other similar foreign agencies is the possibility that the whole picture might be overblown, since heat causes only a very small release of BPAs. On the other hand, studies show measurable levels in the blood of 93 to 98 percent of both young and old people (the older having the higher figure due to the cumulative effect). We should be aware of any accumulating carcinogen since cancer may take many years to develop from repeated "insignificant" exposures. At the time of this writing, some manufacturers of these products have voluntarily banned the use of BPA without waiting for FDA action. It now should be possible for consumers to know if the bottles or food containers they are purchasing are BPA-free, since it is good advertising to make this fact known. Opaque baby-food containers may be already be made of a BPA-free "safe" plastic. After much foot-dragging, the FDA finally banned the use of BPAs in baby bottle production on July 17, 2012. But lo and behold, due to consumer pressure, the industry had already—voluntarily—discontinued using BPA.

SUMMARY

Breast milk, designed for human consumption, is the best possible food for an infant, enabling optimal growth and development. In much of the world there is no alternative. In more "civilized" cultures we have a choice—breast-feeding or artificial-feeding. Our high-paced lifestyle weighs heavily in the decision as to which way to go. Once the mother has carefully considered the pros and cons of both methods—and there are medical conditions which make nursing unfeasible—living with bottle-feeding should be accepted without reservation if that is the choice that is made.

Makers of infant formulas and foods have used the breast-feeding schedule and breast milk nutrition as their benchmark. These "runner-up" products are quite satisfactory; especially those that have been altered the least. Always look at the "ingredients" labels for question-able new additives. "Organic" is best.

As solid foods are blended in to the diet, the older infant and tod-dler will benefit from the added value of the unseen aspects of these new foods, such as the antioxidants in deeply colored fruits and veg-etables, vitamins, and fiber. Just experiencing new foods prepares the infant for acceptance of "grown-up" food when they have the teeth to do their own food grinding.

Another feeding decision for parents to make is weighing the health benefits against the toxic effects of eating fish. There will be more on both of these subjects in our chapter on environmental hazards.

We have tried to help you weigh the advantages of natural and organic foods against their cost and availability, and to see if less expensive substitutes can be made with very little compromise in quality. Feeding involves much more than filling tummies. It should be fulfilling (sorry!) for both the giver and the receiver. If it is not, get help right away, the kind that gets both of you back on track.

CHAPTER 6

WELL-BABY (AND CHILD) CHECKUPS

There are two types of visits to the pediatrician: acute care and the "well" visit, and both are necessary. In the past, a checkup included a complete physical exam, evaluation of physical and neurological development, and nutrition advice. It dealt with health solutions that could not be accomplished during a "sick" visit and covered special interest items in the news, such as hype of low-fat diets, sudden infant death syndrome (SIDS), and other scary things. The pediatrician could provide help to the parents of a "problem" child or a strong-willed child; and have age-appropriate discussions with both the patients and parent(s). These services can't be done in an acute care visit, and much of it has been subtly displaced by the current emphasis on shot clinics and parenting classes that pay little attention to personal, innate "mothering." I see a distinct difference between the one-on-one (one doctor–one family) visits and these newer, almost "production style" clinics.

From the start I want to clarify what I mean by "pediatrician." The medical establishment recognizes pediatricians as only those who have gone through a two-year pediatric residency program and have passed written and oral examinations to achieve "Board Certification" by the American Academy of Pediatrics. This categorizes the board-certified doctor as a specialist. But any specialty is prone to become too narrow in its scope, too afraid to try methods that differ from the general protocol of fellow specialists. If we think of the concept of "primary care," a pediatrician can have a large number of infants and children under his or her care. Personally, I feel that experience and openness are big qualifying factors for this profession.

WELL-BABY AND -CHILD CLINICS

When a mother's precious little one is screaming from the pain of an earache and the doctor is assessing what must be done to provide relief—not only of the unnerving evidence of pain, but of the underlying condition—there is concentrated effort applied to just this one problem. Obviously, this would not be an appropriate time to talk (over the crying) about child development or healthy nutrition. These concerns must be dealt with in the setting of the well-child visit. Rapid changes in the physical development of infants should determine the frequency of these checkups. The closer to birth, the greater the need for more frequent office visits to keep tabs on the rapidly changing infant and to help parents through all kinds of hurdles.

The Well-Baby Examination

The in-house (hospital) examination of a newborn is vital, but there are a great number of adjustments to life in the real world that a newborn makes in the first weeks of life. Coming from the perfect environment of the womb and bursting into the harsh life on the outside taxes the newborn's ability to adapt. That first checkup is vitally important. Abnormal conditions can appear later, under the radar of even the most conscientious and loving parent. An everyday observer (the parent) might not notice subtle day-by-day changes, such as developing anemia or inadequate weight gain. Since the signs of these conditions are cumulative, the experienced provider of a well-check examination can more readily spot them when the infant is seen at intervals.

A complete examination includes not only assessment of all anatomical "parts," but also how they are working. For example, the child's abdomen is examined, but the doctor needs to learn from the parent the nature and frequency of bowel movements. If the doctor finds any hint of deviation from normal after a thorough examination, there will be further questions. The answers will help the pediatrician rule out a disorder or pursue the possibility further. More "quiet" neurological signs such as alertness, eye-following, and muscle tone are assessed, along with age-related developmental landmarks such as head control, appropriate smiling, grasping, rolling over, sitting, crawling, and many more.

In such rapidly developing creatures—the newborns of all mammals—many of the hints of abnormality will disappear by the next doctor visit. On the other hand, some hints may appear stronger on the next visit, and that would require more of a diagnostic workup. The doctor is not hiding the truth by not mentioning why his or her eyebrows rose a little when they first noted something. If the parents have not formed a good doctor-patient relationship yet, or are unduly nervous and lack self-confidence in parenting skills, why add to their anxiety level, especially when a subsequent visit might eliminate the suspicious finding. The only thing gained is more anxiety when testing is prematurely used in an attempt to definitively diagnose.

Nutritional Assessments

Nutrition assessment is much easier with a nursing baby if its mother is healthy. For this reason the "baby" doctor should step out of his role a bit and obtain mother's nutrition history, and talk about both the deficiencies and the necessities for optimal health for her baby. Not only will her baby's nutrition be better assured, but also a good maternal diet, with certain vitamin-mineral supplements, will help the mother counter some of the added strain of nursing, including downright fatigue.

The Value of Well-Baby Visits for Answering General Questions

If this is her firstborn, the mother is bound to have questions concerning feeding, whether by breast or bottle (see infant feeding section for more on this). What should bowel movements look like, and how often can we expect them? How many wet diapers should be expected in twenty-four hours? Crying is an issue likely to raise many questions when there has been no previous experience with a newborn. Medical personnel other than the doctor can provide more help *after* the doctor rules out all out-of-the-ordinary causes that might need further attention. A new, inexperienced mother should never be afraid to ask questions that she sees as valid. There is no such thing as a "dumb" question if it arises from concern. Maternal instincts are powerful. Anything that riles them up should be looked into.

Much of the value of a well-baby or well-child checkup is in the educational opportunities it offers. The fun of a pediatric practice lies both in teaching patients (parents) and learning from them. I always tried to find ways to allow time for this hands-on interchange of ideas. Hand-outs proved helpful—if they were not just handed out. I needed to know that any instructions I gave were fully discussed and understood, even argued, before they were provided. The printed word was just a reminder of our conversation. A busy pediatrician has office personnel trained to do their particular job—from nurses, to physician assistants, to receptionists. Whatever the assigned duties, each person must be well-versed and experienced in his or her particular field, and not afraid to ask someone with more experience about what to do in a special situation. I feel that ancillary personnel can be very helpful and that patients can relate comfortably to them. I also know that sometimes an answer will come from an experience or a bit of seemingly obscure information that I had gained many years before in practice or in medical school.

An infant who refused to eat sparked in me the "crazy" idea that I should look at her eyegrounds (a term describing the area of the retina where the optic nerve emerges). The opthalmoscopic examination revealed signs of a neurologic problem that led to successful removal of a benign tumor near very vital centers in the brain, including one that controls appetite. Surely, after that experience, I didn't check out these specific neurological signs in every infant with poor appetite. I realized that this was a rare condition, and that I should hope I would recognize other rare conditions in the future.

Intraoffice personnel have to be in touch with each another constantly so they can learn from one another. I would greatly prefer to do everything myself, because the detective work is the fun part of diagnosing. One gets clues from the physical examination and the interview of a care giver, forms a working diagnosis, and then proceeds to tear it apart or add to it with tests and more questions. But going it alone is not likely to happen in a busy practice. Any of the office personnel can contribute greatly to a patient's welfare by listening, relating what they hear to their experience, and being willing to say that they don't have the answer but they will try their best to find it. This holds true for the doctor as well. Mutual trust is the key—doctor, office personnel, and patient representative all working together.

Well Clinics Versus Shot Clinics

It is unfortunate that many times *"well" clinics have become shot clinics.* When famous people like Bill Gates (and the Gates Foundation) become convinced that vaccinations will save the children of the world and that lack of money is the only obstacle to a worldwide vaccination program, our federal legislators seem to follow suit.

Lobbyists for vaccine manufacturers have a heyday with the "save the babies of the world" theme (especially in this country). Money is appropriated for individual State Health Departments with mandates of vaccination requirements. Public, county-run well clinics are under the thumb of their respective state's Department of Health and Human Services. The vaccine may be free or of low cost, but county health departments have to comply with the regulations and recommendations for vaccinations, at what age they are given, and which ones to give, in order to obtain them. Private practices are severely affected by these policies, in that this standard of care is set for them. Any deviation could make the "shot giver" subject to a lawsuit. Much effort has to be put into being certain to follow the suggested (or often mandated) state vaccination schedule. As the emphasis on compliance with these regulations increases, the emphasis on the general health perspective of the well visit diminishes. Health clinics become "shot clinics."

The Special Supplemental Nutrition Program for Woman, Infants, and Children (abbreviated as WIC) is a decent federal program designed, along with food stamps, to provide adequate nutrition to the needy. The program works in conjunction with the Department of Agriculture, which determines what foods qualify under the program. They are required to ensure that the issued checks are not used for soft drinks and some processed foods, but it is impossible to completely change established dietary habits with a program such as this. As with vaccination recommendations, nutrition protocol that is provided "from the top" through a federal program can not apply to every individual. WIC often refers infants to government-related well clinics after cursory examinations. The program's intentions are good, but now the infant enters the shot clinic system—the mandated system in which individual needs are not met. A concerned parent should not hesitate to receive all the benefits possible from a system such as this in troubled times. The trick is to learn what is beneficial and what is not. It is much easier to passively accept every service provided, but many of these offerings should be questioned. If they are not questioned, the deficiencies in these programs just roll along unchecked.

"Although most well-child visits for children under three years of age are of 'short duration', parent satisfaction is generally high." This statement came from a cross-sectional national survey that included 1,428 parents, conducted at the University of California, Los Angeles, and published in the October 2011 issue of *Pediatrics*.[1] One-third of these parents reported spending ten minutes or less with "the clinician" (not necessarily a physician); 47 percent reported the visits lasting eleven to twenty minutes. Admittedly, "Longer visits are associated with more developmental screening, discussion of more psychosocial risks and greater parent satisfaction," but in defense of the short visit the results of the survey claimed that "even with the shortest visits parent-reported satisfaction generally was high." In ascertaining why parents were satisfied, "Regardless of the length of the visit 80 percent reported receiving anticipatory guidance on *immunizations* [my emphasis] and breast-feeding with more issues such as sleeping position, feeding issues and car seats being included in the longer visits." Developmental assessment, which formerly was the backbone of the infant well visit, took a back seat to "anticipatory guidance topics" and was done only one-half to two-thirds of the time—more often, of course, in the longer visits.

A decent physical assessment, evaluation of feeding, encouraging questions from parents and answering them, simply cannot be accomplished in ten minutes. If a ten-minute visit is felt to provide satisfaction, it shows that the satisfied parents do not understand what they are missing. It is difficult to prioritize issues that can be squeezed into a ten minute visit. This model will not work either in the public or the private sector. Probably the only way to know whether the pediatrician is going to cover essentials in a well visit is by word of mouth from trusted, like-minded friends.

The Importance of Nutrition and Health Education

Orthomolecular physicians have been using nutrition to treat illness for decades. Mining physicians' reports is immensely valuable: They learned something that we need to know. Health knowledge worth having does not go out of date in seven years or even seventy years. What works is never out of date. This is not hair-splitting. It is an important paradigm: Do what works.

Be cautious of "new lamps for old," as Aladdin learned to be. There has been a great cultural shift. Children are now raised in a world of fast foods, working mothers, television advertising hype, technological advances, and the idea that pharmaceuticals best represent medical science while nutrition therapy doesn't. Made-up syndromes abound, with drug salespeople all too eager to satisfy the created need for "a drug for every ill" whether real or imagined. Symptom relief does not get to root causes. Nutritional medicine can.

Obesity

An overlooked problem I see is that there has been such an acceptance of obesity in infants and children today, partly as a result of dropping the well-visit observation and counsel. Concern and discussion about this problem has been replaced with an "everybody's doing it," "whatever" attitude. So parents buy sloppy, concealing clothes for their kids, who then will be accepted. We make them feel good about themselves to further their "self esteem." Wrong! Being "not with it" is great motivation for the kid (and his parents) who wants to get on the ball. Of course the usual "get off your (shall we say, chair) and play outdoors, rather than with an electronic gadget" comes to mind, and the child might gain some athletic prowess that could help win real friends.

The "well" check can be an important checkpoint for noting an infant who is gaining too much weight so this subtle onset of childhood obesity can be nipped in the bud. Studies have shown that parents are poor judges for estimating normal weight in their children. Also, society's acceptance of obesity has dulled their perception. An outside observer is needed to point this problem out to them. Learning and beginning proper nutrition in infancy will have lifetime rewards.

CHRONIC POOR NUTRITION IN THE UNITED STATES

Only three percent of a large sampling of American adults practices what is commonly considered a healthy lifestyle. An American Medical Association survey of 153,000 men and women between the ages of eighteen and seventy-four found that only 23.3 percent reported consuming five servings of fruits and vegetables per day.[1] The usual U.S. diet provides an insufficient amount of vitamins.[2]

References

1. Reeves, M. J. A. P. Rafferty. "Healthy Lifestyle Characteristics Among Adults in the United States." *Arch Intern Med* 165(8) (Apr 2005):854–857.

2. Fletcher, R. H., K. M. Fairfield. "Vitamins for Chronic Disease Prevention in Adults: Clinical Applications." *JAMA* 287(23) (Jun 19, 2002):3127–3129.

SUMMARY

There have been vast changes in emphasis for well-baby and child checkups—from regular, helpful educational conversations to what we have now: "bytes" of information and lots of shots. What used to work, both in the public and private sector, required a good doctor-patient relationship of *trust* and a good deal of *time*, both of which are lacking today. The push for shots hardly allows for any rebuttal from an informed parent. The office or clinic puts emphasis on whatever predestined topic is in vogue, such as the "back to sleep" program or the safety issues of cribs or strollers. Valuable time that should be used for developmental assessment and nutrition advice is squandered. The change is so well established that it won't be reversed. If a satisfactory alternative cannot be found, separate out the good parts and accept them, but don't feel forced to accept the bad. You can learn of better ways to enhance your infant's health through the references at the end of this book, and by asking friends and professionals you can trust.

CHAPTER 7

MIDDLE EAR INFECTIONS AND OTHER RELATED PROBLEMS

When I moved to Montana in 1970, my first steady job was conducting well-child clinics for the Salish Kootenai tribe. We live on what is called an "open" reservation. It was a closed reservation, but the government opened it up to homesteading. I definitely own my land even though I live on an Indian reservation. The Indian people had access to the same doctors that the rest of us use—through the Indian Health Service. I worked through the service and conducted the clinics. It was at a time when many ear, nose, and throat (ENT) docs were going "ape" over tubes (more on this below), while I was finding an incredible number of milk-allergic kids that got over their ear troubles if they came to my clinic. A group of ENT doctors in nearby Missoula felt business was too slow. They equipped a bus with a surgical suite and toured the territory—literally snatching kids from my clinics. Sometimes they put in ventilation tubes with a child's very first episode of middle ear effusion. This was very disillusioning to me, since I had known some fine ENT docs in my day.

PHYSIOLOGY OF THE EAR

I wonder just how many doctors have been asked by their young charges, "Just where is this middle ear?" I used to have a cut-away model of the anatomy that clearly showed what we were talking about. For now, a word picture will have to do. We see the external ear, a flap on the side of the head, called the pinna. The tunnel of skin heading

PUPPIES, TOO?

A curious sidelight: A number of breeds of dogs are prone to ear infections. I (AWS) found that giving dogs supplemental vitamin C on a regular basis is an effective way to prevent canine ear infections. In my decades of "dogdom," I have observed that vitamin C works for German shepherds, Springer spaniels, and all varieties of mixed breeds. Here is one observation that cannot easily be dismissed as a placebo effect, in that it is somewhat difficult to "psych" a dog into thinking it will not get an ear infection.

for the interior is still part of the external ear until it terminates at the eardrum (tympanic membrane). The cavity behind the drum is the "middle" ear. Further inside is the inner ear. The way this all works to provide hearing is truly amazing.

Sound waves are collected by the shape of the external ear and funneled in toward the eardrum. In order for the eardrum to move, air must be able to escape from the middle ear space. Have you noticed that there is an air hole in the shell of a drum to provide escape for the air? Try plugging the hole while playing the drum. This will greatly dampen the tone. The Eustachian tube provides the necessary ventilation for the air captured in the middle ear. It begins in the middle ear space and opens into the area where the back of the nose enters the throat. Have you ever been able to "pop" your ears open, after an atmospheric pressure change, by holding your nose and gently blowing while swallowing at the same time? That's the result of opening up the Eustachian tube and equalizing the pressure on either side of the eardrum.

The inner ear is even more intriguing. It is a coiled-up, fluid-filled tube with a drumlike membrane at the end, hooked up to the eardrum by means of three little bones. Hair cells of various lengths, which are part of the auditory nerve, project from the tube's inner lining into the liquid. Movement of the drum causes the fluid in the tube to pulse, creating waves that pass over the hair cells like a summer wind over a wheat field. This movement of the hair cells creates a neuroelectric potential in the auditory nerve, which transmits to the auditory receptive area of the brain. The stimulation of the shorter to the longer hair cells provide the perceptions of higher frequency to lower frequency tones.

Exposure to excessive noise level has the effect of causing nerve damage by damaging the hair cells. Higher-frequency sounds are the first to go. Unfortunately, this damage is permanent, so prevention is key. On the other hand, anything that impedes movement of the eardrum or otherwise prevents the mechanical energy transfer from the eardrum to the inner ear is called conduction deafness, and is subject to preventive measures and is responsive to treatment. Essentially, nerve damage is not an issue for infants. They have not had the noise pollution exposure. However, we have to be aware that there are some drugs and antibiotics administered to infants that are capable of causing auditory nerve damage.

The Adenoids

In the area of convergence of the Eustachian tubes on the nasopharynx is the adenoid—an almond-shaped bit of lymphoid tissue like a tonsil—lying between the Eustachian tube openings. We think of lymphoid tissue, like tonsils, as flaring from bacterial infections. Actually most tonsillitis (and adenoiditis) is viral, but we do not want to miss "strep" tonsillitis, which can have a serious aftermath. Allergies can also cause swelling of these lymphoid tissues. Infants are more prone to Eustachian tube dysfunction (blockage) and otitis media (OM) in that there is almost a straight shot (horizontal) from the infant's nasopharynx to the middle ear through a tube that is shorter and of relatively larger caliber than that of an older child. When sinus openings are partially blocked by inflammation, the sinus drainage, or "postnasal drip," is a source of irritation and inflammation of the nasopharynx and Eustachian tube openings.

MIDDLE EAR PROBLEMS

We will speak of middle ear problems as otitis media (OM) although the problem may not have an "itis" (inflammation) component to it.

(And please don't confuse this "OM" with the abbreviation for Ortho-molecular Medicine.)

Middle ear effusions develop quietly and don't produce an earache. Momentary discomfort from a "stopped up" Eustachian tube is relieved as described below. The real pain comes from an acute middle ear infection.

Middle Ear Infections

Let's first deal with a middle ear infection, in which puslike material is formed in the middle ear space. Acute otitis media is still the major reason for emergency care in infancy and early childhood.[1] Why? Because it often creates an earache. (If you have ever experienced an earache, I would bet that you could recall the incident even if it occurred at a very young age, due to the intense discomfort.) But why is this such a common affliction?

Humans carry all kinds of disease-causing bacteria in our noses and throats that may enter the middle ear space. The bad bugs might be there without causing harm to the host, in which case the person is a "carrier." This status changes when there is an obstruction that prevents access to air and interferes with the drainage of normal secretions. Whether the blockage is caused by a virus infection, bacterial infection, allergy, or irritant, whatever bacteria are in, or move into, the middle ear will flourish. As pressure builds from pus formation, pain intensifies.

Most middle ear infections that show signs of both inflammation and fluid in the middle ear, and cause immobility of the eardrum, are of viral etiology. There are subtle signs that can tell the examiner that it is a primary or secondary bacterial infection instead. Unfortunately, many times, a careful diagnostic examination is not done, and the parent, who doesn't know any better, might convince the doctor (who *should* know better) to prescribe an antibiotic. Physicians have been warned for decades not to succumb to this pressure, but it is still prevalent. Consequently, we are in a mess due to bacterial resistance to commonly used antibiotics. Studies performed in countries with public healthcare that enables a "free" doctor visit support waiting on antibiotic coverage until there can be a follow-up visit with another examination. If there is a change in the infant's overall condition, such as recurring pain or fever, the doctor should be notified sooner, but generally the problem clears after several weeks, and the length of time is similar in the two groups (those taking antibiotics versus those that don't). In the United States, insurance providers are not likely to reimburse the doctor for a follow-up visit, so antibiotic coverage is provided "just in case." Thus, the potential for developing a chronic condition and/or antibiotic resistance continues.

What to Do

The first step to solving a middle ear problem is an examination that searches for clinical signs of infection. A check of the nose, throat, ears, and associated lymph nodes in the neck helps determine what could be causing a middle ear problem. Just seeing a bloodshot eardrum is not significant when the surrounding tissues are showing the same clinical sign. If the eardrum is bulging and, particularly, if this is accompanied with fever, that spells infection. At this point it must be determined whether the infection is bacterial or viral. If there is little sign of infection but the drum appears dull, or if an older child doesn't seem to be hearing well, we are dealing with a more chronic condition. The examiner can also use another useful diagnostic tool, the pneumo-otoscope. The mobility of the eardrum can be checked by alternately squeezing and releasing a rubber bulb attached by a tube to the body of the otoscope. If it doesn't move, some kind of material is in the middle ear space and hearing can be drastically reduced. If the material has been there for some time, a "glue ear" may have developed that will need further attention.

An infant's cry for help when he or she is suffering an earache is unnerving for parent and doctor alike. When I saw the eardrum was bulging and dull, I knew that pressure from infection caused the pain. And as brutal as it might sound, I obtained full agreement from the parent, after a thorough explanation, to proceed with a myringotomy. In a myringotomy a topical anesthesia, in the form of drops to the eardrum, is applied. An incision is then made into the bulging drum with a small sharp blade, through the speculum of the otoscope. An almost immediate cessation of crying follows the release of the infected fluid and consequent relief of pressure. The other satisfying aspect of this surgical treatment is the knowledge that any sort of abscess (walled-off infection) clears much faster after surgical drainage. It is difficult for an antibiotic to get to an abscess through the bloodstream.

EASING EARACHES THE HOMESTEADER'S WAY

When I (AWS) learned that many medicines for earache are actually ineffective, even though still commonly prescribed, I realized that I was going to have to find alternatives. Back in 1983, the *New England Journal of Medicine* reported that a three-year study of decongestants and antihistamines commonly prescribed by ear specialists showed that they are no better than nothing at all.[1] Putting tubes in a child's ears is hardly a pleasing alternative. When your child (toddler, older child, or even an adult family member) has pain in or around the ear, here are some other approaches that may help:

1. Simple earache is likely to be a symptom of an ear infection. Almost anything you do to fight the infection will fight the earache as well. Large doses of vitamin C are especially effective. At high levels, vitamin C is a natural antibiotic and antihistamine. It will also reduce inflammation and fever, and is safer than pharmaceutical drugs. The books listed below will substantiate and elaborate on this, and are very important for you to read.

2. Check and see where the pain is. It might be external. To check this out, find the place where the neck, skull, and jaw meet. This spot is just under the ear. If gentle pressure on this spot is painful, you may have a tender lymph node. This node flares with other types of pharyngitis (throat inflammation). It is worth asking your doctor, or reading up on the subject, to find out which.

3. Warm, damp compresses are a traditional earache treatment. A washcloth moistened in warm tap water works fine and feels good.

Even better is vitamin E oil, introduced carefully into the ear canal. My kids found this to be very soothing.

4. To help relieve pressure and encourage natural drainage, you can try a simple massage technique. *Gently* press right under each ear. Now continue *gently* pressing, moving downward and forward along and just under the edge of the jawbone. You have just massaged the muscles and pharyngeal area near the Eustachian tubes, those internal passages described earlier that connect the inside of each ear to its own opening in the upper throat. Repeatedly massaging like this aids in relaxing the entire region and often helps reduce ear-area discomforts. If the child shows a pain response, stop. Before resorting to artificial tubes, let's try the ones we were born with.

5. I, like a lot of health nuts, believe that earaches and infections are fundamentally caused by improper diet. Sometimes allergy is the problem and milk is the culprit. Many kids are fed generous quantities of meat, white bread, sugar, and junk food daily. This must stop, or the earaches won't. I think that a plant-based diet with lots of fruit, vegetable salads, whole grains, beans and legumes, nuts, and other non-meat protein results in healthier children. Think that your kids won't accept these good foods?

Consider the useless fallback of pharmaceutical medicines, which are often no better than a placebo. Start your children eating right early, and it will pay dividends for a lifetime.

The above really seemed to work for my family, especially the high-dose vitamin C. My children were raised without a single dose of antibiotic, ever. The only time my kids ever saw a doctor was for a physical.

References

1. Cantekin, E. I., E. M. Mandel, C. D. Bluestone, et al. "Lack of Efficacy of a Decongestant-Antihistamine Combination for Otitis Media with Effusion (Secretory Otitis Media) in Children—Results of a Double-Blind, Randomized Trial." *New Eng J Med* 308(6) (Feb 10, 1983):297–301.

Recommended Reading

Hickey, S., A. W. Saul. *Vitamin C: The Real Story*. Laguna Beach, CA: Basic Health, 2008.

Pauling, L. *How To Live Longer and Feel Better*. 20th anniversary edition. Corvallis, OR: Oregon State University Press, 2006.

Smith, L. H. *Clinical Guide to the Use of Vitamin C: The Clinical Experiences of Frederick R. Klenner, M.D.* Portland, OR: Life Sciences Press, 1988. Adapted from: *Vitamin C as a Fundamental Medicine: Abstracts of Dr. Frederick R. Klenner, M.D.'s Published and Unpublished Work*. Reprinted 1991. Available online at http://www.whale.to/a/smith_b.html (accessed April 2013).

Stone, I. The Healing Factor: Vitamin C Against Disease. New York: Grosset & Dunlap, 1972.

Once the situation is less frenetic—after pain is relieved or during a follow-up well check—it is important that the physician try to discover what is going on in the family setting. Predisposing causes should be considered, such as head colds and other upper respiratory virus infections, home interior renovating with noxious substances in the air, a past history of nasal allergy related to an off and on stuffy nose, or consistent mouth-breathing due to adenoid obstruction.

Treatment for Middle Ear Problems

Clearing the nasal secretions that periodically develop during a cold by using a nasal syringe is helpful, but may not be enough to avoid problems. A humidifier will help keep secretions loose if the child's room air is heated and dry. Giving water between regular feedings may be helpful. Saline drops moisten the nasal membranes and thin secretions.

I recommend the *short-term* use (no more than three days) of a pediatric nose drop, especially if ear troubles are recurring. Clear the nose as well as you can, and then place no more than two drops in each nostril in the morning, at midday, and particularly at bedtime. There is no danger if you follow these directions, but there certainly is danger in long-term use of these products. These medicines are vasoconstrictors, which relieve swelling of the tissues they are applied to. General vaso-constriction can result in a rise in blood pressure if too much is assimilated. Certainly, there is no danger in using small amounts short-term in a pediatric drop preparation. Nose drops get their bad reputation because of people who didn't heed the warnings on the adult preparations and became dependent on the drops for obtaining any kind of a normal airway after weeks of use. Laborious weaning is required to get back to easy nose breathing. A test to determine whether the nasal airway is open enough in an infant is done by taking a wisp of cotton and putting it in the front of the airstream, one nostril at a time, of the sleeping baby. Look for movement caused by the breeze. At the time of this writing, I could not find any nose drops suitable for infant use on the over-the-counter shelf. I hope one of these useful preparations will reappear. If not, just diligently employ the other measures for clearing the nasal airway.

Antibiotic Use for Middle Ear Infections

The rise of bacterial antibiotic resistance caused by antibiotic overuse means that careful consideration must be given to deciding which, if any, antibiotic is to be prescribed for an infant or young child. The decision as to whether it is safe to wait a few days to see if there is spontaneous improvement, risking the possible danger of a rapid spread of infection that can cause mastoiditis (infection in the surrounding spongy bone) or meningitis (infection of the covering of the brain that lies adjacent to the mastoid), is a weighty one. Both bacterial and viral infections can produce a "gunky" (for lack of a good medical word) discharge, as white cells fighting infection are sacrificed on the battlefield. Even considering other means of differentiating viral from bacterial disease, there is no 100 percent certainty as to the cause. A more symptomatic infection—accompanied by pain, fever, obvious inflammation, a bulging eardrum—will most likely push the decision to antibiotic therapy.

Any infection should be followed up with another examination to make sure it has been completely eliminated, because without a complete resolution there will be some degree of hearing impairment. Our current medical care system often does not cover a follow-up visit—a fact that sways the physician to "cover" himself by providing an antibiotic prescription "just in case." Rather than guessing what organism is causing the infection or what antibiotic will take care of it, the health professional should check with the local hospital laboratory to see what organisms are prevalent in the community and to find out their antibiotic resistance or susceptibility. Whether or not an antibiotic is prescribed, parents should request a follow-up visit to be certain the problem is resolved.

OM WITH EFFUSION

Less dramatic but equally important is the presence of fluid in the middle ear space, as it indicates *Eustachian tube dysfunction*. I have never felt that this is an appropriate term. How can the ventilation tube function (ventilate) when it is blocked or when air in the middle ear space is replaced with fluid? If it is clear, it functions just fine. I think the medical terminology for chronic middle ear effusion, "glue ear"—even though it sounds like a lay term—is very apt. If the middle-ear space has inadequate drainage and is shut off from fresh air, bacteria will multiply rapidly and increase the pressure and resultant pain. If there is no infection but a blockage is present because the tissues surrounding the tube opening are swollen, there may be no pain but there will be inevitable hearing loss—not so easy to detect in an infant. The longer the fluid remains trapped, the more gluelike it becomes (a process called inspissation) as the more liquid portion is absorbed. The eardrum will appear dull. A more accurate assessment can be made with an instrument that measures eardrum mobility (described above). If it can't move, it won't do its job.

A search for the cause of this condition should be made after even the first episode. It will probably first be detected at a follow-up visit for an acute middle ear infection that reveals incomplete resolution. I have found nasal allergy from food allergens (commonly cow's milk sensitivity) or inhalants (such as second-hand tobacco smoke) to be the most common predisposing factors in chronic OM with effusion in infants.

Food Allergies

Food allergies can create swelling in the mucous membranes of the nose and throat in much the same way as inflammation from infection or inhaled irritants. In infants, the most common food allergen of all is cow's milk. (This makes a good case, but not a perfect one, for breast-feeding.) Rarely, if there is milk in the mother's diet, undigested cow's milk protein can sneak into mother's bloodstream and be secreted into her breast milk, sensitizing her infant. I had two infants under my care (at different times) of a mother who pulled off this more rare manifestation of cow's milk allergy. The first time this happened it was puzzling to figure out what the problem was. The second time was easy. All we had to do was take cow's milk out of the mother's diet and substitute it with other foods to cover her nutrition needs.

Allergy Symptoms

An allergic nose is an itchy nose. Even young infants can figure out a way to rub their noses without using their hands. And infants exhibiting nasal allergy symptoms are likely to show signs of gastroenteral distress (what scientific medicine calls *tummy ache* [or TA, but only in the most sophisticated pediatric journals]).

Traditional Medical Treatments

Instead of trying to achieve normal function of our built-in ventilation tubes, a surgical procedure to detour around a blocked Eustachian tube began to grow in popularity at least forty-five years ago. A small plastic tube, called a ventilation tube, was introduced into the middle ear through an incision (myringotomy) in the eardrum (the procedure is called a tympanoplasty). Any fluid present was sucked out prior to insertion of the tube—a tough procedure in itself if the child had "glue ear." The end of the tube was barbed so it would be more likely to remain in place. There was no question that the procedure helped, whether from cleaning out the middle ear space or by providing enough ventilation so the eardrum could move a bit. However, there were no studies I was aware of that compared a more conservative treatment with this surgical approach. I did my own study of my patients, all of whom were children receiving nonsurgical treatment. I had probably over one hundred "controls" of infants and children, and I made certain that hearing was brought back to normal. In the case of infants, eardrum movement and appearance had to be normal at the end of their treatment. "Conservative treatment" was simply identifying and relieving the underlying causes of their problem. I was fortunate to have a conservative ENT doctor to consult with if I felt the need. He performed an adenoidectomy on several of the patients I referred to him, but he did not use ventilation tube insertion.

I have one anecdote that supported my view that there were other ways "to skin the cat." As one of the breast-fed, milk-allergy boys (see above) grew up, he fell off the wagon and reverted to imbibing cow's milk again. When he complained of not hearing well, the embarrassed parents couldn't face my wrath and went to another doctor. The boy was promptly referred for placement of tubes. Later, the wayward son had an earache, and his parents noted that creamy liquid was exuding from one ear canal. They swallowed their pride and allowed me to examine him. Sure enough, puslike fluid was exiting the middle ear *through the intact ventilation tube.*

There is another mainstream form of medical treatment for middle ear problems that I used at first, before I really thought about it: prophylactic (supposedly preventive) antimicrobial medication for chronic effusion. Initially, a sulfa drug was used for this treatment, which was replaced later by an antibiotic. Sulfa drugs are more prone to cause sensitization reactions—some of them serious. And antibiotics used in this way can become useless as the bacteria become resistant. The short time I tried this preventive program, I found it accomplished little prevention and no "cures," compared to getting at the root causes.

VITAMIN C FOR MIDDLE EAR INFECTIONS

All infants need proper nutrition including a daily multiple vitamin. Those prone to middle ear infection or effusion need extra vitamin C, which should be started with *any* sign of nasal congestion. It is possible but not easy to find a good, inexpensive vitamin C preparation in an easy-to-administer form. We suggest that you make your own. You can do this, since an overdose is hard to achieve, and precision is not vital. The most practical way to get supplemental vitamin C into a child is by stirring 1,000 mg (one-quarter teaspoon) of vitamin C crystals (powder) into a small amount of fruit juice. (We will return to this in the vitamin C chapter.) Plain water works fine to dissolve the vitamin C, but plain water fails to enhance your chances of getting it into the youngster. Make it easy for everyone concerned: Use the child's very favorite fruit juice to make success more likely. Keep this solution refrigerated; vitamin C deteriorates with heat. If crystals settle out of the liquid, shake it before using. Since vitamin C is water soluble and the body is constantly excreting it out, it is better to divide the total daily dose to make three or four doses throughout the waking hours. For an older baby of twenty pounds, anywhere in a range of 50 to 500 mg per dose would be appropriate. That is not a lot: 500 mg is one-eighth of a teaspoon of pure vitamin C powder, and 50 mg is a tiny amount; a tenth of and an eighth of a teaspoon, respectively. Use your baby's weight as your rough guide. Do not get hung up on the dosage details. Look for the individual amount that helps your baby relieve stuffiness. The effective dose is the effective dose. We are not playing word games here: All children and situations are different. Take enough C to be symptom free, whatever that amount might be. How do you know if you gave too much? You get to "bowel tolerance," which means exactly what you think it means. Back off a bit if the baby's bowels become a bit loose or the child is flatulent. Again, in this mathematically correct era, it is almost counterintuitive to say that the vitamin dose is not fixed. Well, it isn't. *There is no set amount.* It depends on need. As you can be confident that you will do no harm, give the amount that works.

CHAPTER 8

COLDS, INFLUENZA, AND OTHER RESPIRATORY ILLNESSES

Nobody likes a baby to get sick, and that includes the baby. Although not serious, the common cold in an infant is a more than just a nuisance. It is a challenge to keep him or her comfortable and free of complications. Influenza and other virus respiratory infections can turn nasty. "Strep" (a bacterial) infection has also been included in this chapter, which is organized on a from-bad-to-worse basis.

THE COMMON COLD

The "common cold" affects the tip-top of the respiratory tree. Since the term "common cold," which describes both its causes and signs, sounds entirely too common for those of us in the medical field, we professionals use some more satisfying "medicalese" synonyms instead: nasopharyngitis (inflammation in the area where the back of the nose enters the throat) and acute coryza (runny nose and eyes), caused most commonly by a rhinovirus (think of a *rhino*ceros with a horn for a nose). The usage of the word "cold" comes from a centuries-old, still controversial concept that a cold follows exposure to cold temperatures, or having suffered from a chill. I see no problem with this ancient concept when thinking of disease brought about by both an agent (a virus) and a susceptible victim with its defenses down—in this case the victim being an immune system stressed from cold exposure. Of course, one can also "catch a cold" without having suffered cold stress.

The cold starts, usually two or three days after exposure to the virus, with a runny nose and a scratchy throat that can develop into a sore throat. There may be sneezing and what I call a hacky or "dumb" dry cough emanating from an irrepressible tickle in the throat. There are often muscle aches, chilling, and malaise (feeling weak, depressed, and just plain awful). There may even be a low-grade fever at the cold's onset. These symptoms usually diminish after the first two days. Meanwhile the nasal secretions can thicken and become pretty "gunky," which causes much distress in an infant. Infants do not like detouring around the nose and having to mouth breathe.

Treatment

When treating an infant or toddler for a common cold, consider the usual types of treatment used for discomfort from aches and difficulty breathing through the nose (we presume infants are like big people in this respect). Consider whether a low fever should be treated for the fever itself, or if it is just that the fever is part of what is also creating a headache, muscle aches, or general misery. There are sections in this book describing fever treatment and over-the-counter medications in more detail. Keep in mind that there is little or no place for the use of most of these preparations in infants. Keeping the airway as clear as possible should be our first priority in a cold remedy, since obstruction can lead to secondary infection in the middle ear or, more rarely, in the underdeveloped infant nasal sinuses. Let's deal with these items, one by one.

It is best to avoid medicine for fever or presumed other discomforts if the cold is not complicated by a secondary infection and the infant is not terribly fussy. At last, the use of antipyretics (fever reducers) and painkillers such as acetaminophen, ibuprofen, (and formerly) aspirin in infants is coming under scrutiny. These products are terribly misused because of misleading advertising. In short, there are more "cons" than "pros" to the use of these substances, and the effectiveness to risk ratio is not favorable. For now, let us look for other ways to deal with the miseries of a cold.

Keep the nasal airway as clear as possible, especially at bedtime to aid sleep. The inflammation and mucus production in the nasopharynx will predispose the child toward middle ear infection and coughing. Learn to use a nasal aspirator, a device for drawing mucus out of the nose. It consists of a glass or plastic tube with a blunt tip on one end and a stiff rubber bulb on the other. To use it, squeeze the air out of the bulb with your fingers, and keep this pressure on the bulb while you place the tip on the other end firmly into a nostril. Once the tip is in place, release the finger pressure on the bulb and allow it to expand. The vacuum this causes will pull mucus out of the nasal passage. The nice thing about the transparent end is that you can see results.

After a day or two, when the mucus is thicker—thousands of white blood cells have laid down their lives as they fought the infection, creating the more viscous "gunk"—aspiration may need some help. Saline of normal, non-irritating concentration is available in drug stores and supermarkets. A homemade preparation is also acceptable, and can be administered with a soft rubber syringe or a blunt-tipped medicine dropper. Make a solution of one-quarter teaspoon of table salt in eight ounces of lukewarm water. Place the infant in a semi-reclining position, put in a few drops, and immediately try to aspirate the thinned-out mucus and debris. Allow a toddler to have a preview of what is going to happen. He can even taste the saline that will eventually make its way into his throat. The aspirator can be tested on the back of the hand or by drawing water from a glass. Of course, no aspirator is necessary if he can master the difficult art of nose blowing.

I found membrane-shrinking nose drops (of pediatric strength) to be very useful at bedtime when nasal aspiration and saline drops just did not suffice. However, in 2007, the FDA warned against using them and in 2008 manufacturers stopped making them. The problem was overuse. The FDA said that "reports of harm occurred when the child received too much medication such as in cases as accidental ingestion, unintentional overdose, or after a medication dosing error."[1] This type of preparation had often been abused, leading to dependency in order to allow any air to pass through the nasal airway. I feel that a careful parent, who knows what is going on, will not allow any of these possible causes of harm to take place. One last aid might be in the form of using a humidifier, near the bedside, at night.

The best medicine, not only for symptom relief but for truly fighting the infection, is vitamin C. It must be emphasized that no tangible results will be seen if you use the small amounts usually suggested for infants. The general rule of "bowel tolerance" can be safely applied to infants just as well as it is for adults. Remember that bowel tolerance indicates saturation of vitamin C. We are not advocating diarrhea; bowel tolerance refers to loose stool or flatulence. You may be able to find a convenient form of liquid vitamin C for infants.

Homemade vitamin C solution can be made with powdered or crystalline ascorbic acid, which is generally available in a potency of 1,000 milligrams (mg) per one-quarter teaspoon. Sometimes the crystalline form runs higher, at 1,250 mg per one-quarter teaspoon; some vitamin C powders are lower strength with only half that. Read the label—always, always, always. One teaspoonful, or 4,000 mg when added to five ounces of orange juice or lemonade (thirty teaspoonfuls), will provide thirty doses of about 125 mg each. Being water-soluble, vitamin C should be given in divided doses—start with 125 mg (1 teaspoonful of liquid) three times a day. For a toddler, start with 250 mg, three times a day. Store the solution in the refrigerator, but stir it each time since some of the powder or crystals may settle. Dissolved vitamin C loses punch with time, so recharge the solution once a week with another half-teaspoon or so. The juice should make the solution sufficiently palatable for an infant, but if not, sweeten the deal. A pinch of sugar can be added to the individual dose if your baby grimaces from the sour vitamin C. You also have the option, discussed elsewhere in this book, of using calcium ascorbate. Calcium ascorbate is vitamin C, is available in powder form, and is nonacidic. It is also more expensive and somewhat harder to find in health food stores, but it is easy to obtain on the Internet. Either way, if the dose tolerated well, increase the amount by a half-teaspoon per dose at a time, until you notice that the stools are looser than before. If this occurs, back off. This is what is meant by bowel tolerance. (We repeat this because it is so important . . . and so handy.)

VITAMIN C IS THE KEY

High-dose vitamin C is a known booster for immune system function. If you have not yet looked at Dr. Robert F. Cathcart's website http://www.orthomed.com (or http://vitamincfoundation.org/www.orthomed.com/), you don't know what you are missing. It is exactly what parents want and need: a medical doctor's explanation coupled with tons of information on the antibiotic, antiviral, antitoxin, and antihistamine properties of vitamin C in huge (that is to say, effective) doses.

Should Dr. Cathcart's website be taken down, an internet search for his name will find alternate postings of his work.

Some other sites with information of interest include:

Dr. Cathcart's comments on pH-neutral sodium ascorbate intravenous vitamin C at http://www.vitamincfoundation.org/docc.html.

Instructions written by Dr. Cathcart to tell your doctor precisely how to make up a vitamin C IV solution: http://www.doctoryourself.com/ vit-civ.html.

Parents facing serious illness should read this straight away: "How to Get Intravenous Vitamin C Given to a Hospitalized Patient: An Intravenous Vitamin C Checklist" posted at: http://www.doctoryourself .com/strategies.html. Highly experienced vitamin C specialist Robert F. Cathcart, M.D., has personally endorsed these guidelines, writing: "Thank you so much for this. I think it is great. I am linking to your article on my website."

WORSE "COLDS"

There are many other virus agents that can cause cold symptoms and more: influenza, parainfluenza, respiratory syncytial virus (RSV), adenoviruses, and even some enteroviruses, which cause, primarily, intestinal upsets. We should not lump these together with the common cold. While several share the same cold symptoms, each virus creates its different expression of signs and symptoms in its more severe form. During the course of an illness caused by one of these viruses, the first days after onset produce signs and symptoms indistinguishable from the common cold. The illness might remain at this milder level or develop to a more specific and severe show of signs and symptoms. The potent RSV, which some say is as common as the rhinovirus as a causative agent of illness in young children, may remain a mild cold or evolve rapidly into bronchiolitis, the severe disease described below.

Influenza

Influenza, commonly known as the flu, has some characteristic signs with some variation each year. The "cold" signs are exaggerated. The chill and fever are stronger and higher than with a normal cold. The throat grows more sore. The cough becomes harder and more persistent. It is the headache and muscle aches that are so much worse. A typical flu headache feels like it is centered in the eyes or just above. It may feel like the scalp itself hurts. It is accentuated with every cough. Muscle aches can be severe.

It is usually several days before the fever and aches and pains let up. At this time the cough may become productive and frontal sinuses begin to drain (revealing that the aching eyeballs were from frontal sinus congestion). After the fever breaks, there follows a period of below-normal body temperature associated with feeling really low—*very* low in body, mind, and spirit. At the same time sinus congestion lessens and bronchial secretions loosen, leading to a cough that sounds worse but is far better than the dry hack. I (RKC) am assuming that the adult model I have described is also somewhat expressed in the infant. In some epidemics, intestinal upset is prominent, more commonly so in infants and young children. In recent years I have seen a trend of nausea and intestinal upset playing a bigger part of the symptom complex.

Referring to personal experience and conversation with other adults, I find that, that with an influenza infection, one feels better when running a fever, even a substantial fever, as opposed to "feeling like a truck ran over me" during the low period after the fever breaks. The infant's only way to express his or her misery might be to cry. There is reason to believe that lowering fever with medicines might dampen a healthy immune response. As with a cold, I would treat with medicine only when other means of controlling a high fever were inadequate, and as a way to aid nighttime sleeping. As with any time a baby is sick, feedings and offerings of water may need to be smaller and more frequent, to assure decent nutrition and hydration. (Nursing babies will self regulate regarding their need for food and water.) Infants usually don't cough much. A better indication of the need for a humidifier will be the thickness of nasal secretions. Of course, attention should be paid to setbacks, noted by another rise in fever, fussiness, or just plain not being "normal"—that might indicate secondary infection and a need to be checked out by your doctor.

Advice for prevention and treatment of influenza in infants, unfortunately, has been terribly muddied. Every year, medical bodies such as the American Academy of Pediatrics (AAP), the Centers for Disease Control and Prevention (CDC) or even a higher authority, the World Health Organization (WHO) recommend providing influenza immunization to younger and younger children and infants. Yet, there are virtually no studies regarding the efficacy of the vaccine—that compare the incidence of influenza in vaccinated infants (or other age groups, for that matter) with that in a similar unvaccinated population. Influenza vaccines have had their share of bad effects. Physicians are pushed by the standards laid down by these higher medical authorities. Many feel they cannot challenge them—which makes for a very difficult situation for an informed parent. But if one infant, whose parent talked the doctor out of demanding the shot, had a complicated course from an influenza infection, he or she could be in a lot of trouble. These matters are further discussed in the immunization chapter.

There are indications that the status of the immune system in both vaccinated and unvaccinated individuals is a big factor in both susceptibility and severity of influenza. There is clear evidence that a high degree of prevention can be obtained from high doses of vitamin D. This knowledge is rapidly expanding since the wonders of vitamin D are being accepted by mainstream medicine. There have been many studies about vitamin D and immune health in children and adults but none, so far, in infants. During "flu" season, I recommend 800 International Units (IU) of vitamin D each day, which could be a normal daily recommendation. (I use quotes around flu here, since I feel the word "flu" trivializes the concept of influenza. Years ago, I noted the way parents under my care tossed the word "flu" around. I had my receptionist ask them what they meant by "flu." About half of a large number thought it referred to a vomiting-diarrhea illness. I tried through public announcements to set the record straight.)

The suggested increases of vitamin D dosage recommendations for infants are relatively new, so we should all keep abreast of current recommendations.

Croup

Croup, the common name for laryngotracheobronchitis, is most notable for inflammation of the larynx, as it produces hoarseness and a cough that sounds like a seal bark (in a toddler, not in an infant). A little inflammation goes a long way toward restricting the small airway of an infant. With an increase in swelling, obstruction to the intake of air is noted by the sounds of stridor (noisy inspiration) and a high-pitched wheezing sound on expiration. As stridor increases, a sinking in, or depression, might be seen below the sternum (breast bone) and the drawing in of each breath may cause retraction between the ribs.

The disease process usually stops with mild stridor and the bark-like cough, but it can progress to the point of causing marked distress. An infant becomes fussier; a toddler might want to be more upright in bed. The sides of the nostrils are seen to flare as if trying to provide a larger airway. If the involvement of infection is mainly in the larynx, duration of the croup is shorter. If bronchi are more heavily involved, the croup is of longer duration and may show signs of bronchospasm (a constriction of the muscles of the bronchi) and trouble getting air out of the lungs (wheezing).

Parainfluenza virus accounts for about three-quarters of cases of croup, with the other viruses mentioned above (including measles) accounting for the rest. Of the three strains of parainfluenza virus, one seems more responsible for fall episodes of croup and another for spring outbreaks. Some more severe forms are caused by bacterial infections and should respond to appropriate antibiotic therapy. Any real difficulty breathing needs professional attention. Croup often starts with cold symptoms for one or two days before larynx involvement. For some, the larynx seems to be a weak spot for a respiratory infection—something that runs in the family—leading to repeated bouts of croup in the first five years of life.

Treatment

When an older infant or toddler is having problems breathing, he or she can pick up on a parent's anxiety and worsen the condition. Air will pass through the swollen lining of the larynx and trachea more easily if breathing is relaxed. There is no place for panic. Understanding what is going on is reassuring, as is seeing improvement through treatment.

The little patient will breathe easier in an upright position. So, a useful remedy is to get a hot, hard-running shower bouncing off the shower floor and converting the bathroom into a sauna. A few minutes in the steam, along with soothing reassurances, should relieve the spasm of croup. A humidifier by the bed will help the process continue. Liquids and vitamin C are the only effective "medicines." I have found that grapefruit juice is a good expectorant ("loosener-upper" of thick secretions) for a toddler. A bout of croup usually has the acute (noisy) phase for only one night (yes, night, as in "the middle of the") and then it tapers off. But increasing trouble breathing deserves close attention. In rare cases, the airway can become greatly compromised and require emergency care. Professional evaluation can define whether simple, added treatment will suffice or whether a more serious infection is underway. If airway obstruction is too severe, the physician in the emergency room setting has a useful tool at his disposal. An adrenaline derivative, in mist form, can be put directly on the laryngeal tissues by means of a positive pressure machine. This produces a fast, dramatic improvement. If the child is sick enough to need a physician's attention, evaluation can be made as to whether the croup is brought on by the more rare bacterial infection (usually *H. influenzae*).

Epiglottitis

This overwhelming condition is most commonly due to a bacterial infection from *H. influenzae*. Infants seem to be spared this condition, but it hits children in the two- to seven-year-old range. A progression of croup symptoms is extremely rapid. Fever is a more prominent part of the infection than it is in simple croup. Obstructed breathing causes alarming signs and an obvious need for emergency care.

Typically, shortly after awakening at night, the child shows signs of respiratory distress, but also exhibits an inability to speak and can be seen drooling. He will prefer to be upright, and the older child might want to lean forward as if trying to straighten out his airway. The epiglottis is the trapdoor, or flap valve, that covers the larynx (voice box) when swallowing to prevent breathing in whatever is in the mouth. If it is swollen from infection, the speaking voice will sound muffled at first. With more inflammation, even saliva does not go down easily. The presence of these signs means *get immediate emergency care.*

Treatment

Even professionals looking for an inflamed epiglottis (it looks like a cherry behind the base of the tongue) must proceed cautiously. Carelessly depressing the tongue with a tongue blade could create gagging and spasm that would cause complete blockage of the airway. Other means of observation, such as a lateral view x-ray, may be needed. With the child in this condition, equipment and skilled personnel are on standby to provide an emergency airway if necessary.

Clinical signs may add up sufficiently to make an accurate diagnosis when the child is in this critical state, and it is possible to proceed with an appropriate antibiotic. More important, a super-potent cortisone derivative injection is given to quell the swelling and relieve respiratory distress until the antibiotic has a chance to work (twelve to twenty-four hours).

Strep Tonsillitis

Tonsillitis is right up there with otitis media as a reason for a doctor visit at either the office . . . or the emergency room. Symptoms can hardly be noticed in infants, who can't express themselves. The older the child, the more the similarities there will be to adult signs and symptoms. The point is, it is appropriate to rely more on even gut feelings that the little one is sick. (I hope busy parents don't lose the art of motherhood, including some of the wonderful animal-like instincts.)

Tonsillitis is as the name implies—inflammation of the tonsils. The tonsils reside, one on each side, back near the base of the tongue. The uvula is like a stalactite in the middle. Tonsils are big aggregates of lymphoid tissue that work in behalf of our immune defense. There are smaller patches of lymphoid tissue in a ring that includes tissue at the base of the tongue, the adenoid in the center (which can block the nasal airway), and even in the back of the throat. In a person with nasal allergy who has had the adenoid and tonsils surgically removed, the remaining patches enlarge as if to show that this protective tissue will not completely surrender its duty.

Many bouts of tonsillitis are due to a virus infection, but more attention has to be paid when it is caused by *Streptoccocus pyogenes* (the current name for "strep"). *Pyogenes* implies "pus producing." This group A Streptococcus bacterium can cause strep tonsillitis (pharyngo-tonsillitis) and other acute inflammatory diseases, such as tonsillar abscesses and impetigo. A toxin produced by this group can cause scarlet fever and make one truly sick. Strep throat and tonsillitis usually manifest with fever, sore throat, swollen and tender lymph nodes, and even foul breath. In other words, this illness needs attention.

Two serious diseases can come as an aftermath of a strep infection: rheumatic fever, which bites the heart valves, and glomerulonephritis, which affects the kidneys. During my medical training and pediatric residency training I saw many victims of rheumatic fever. About twenty days after an untreated (by penicillin) group A strep infection, long after the acute symptoms of strep throat have subsided, very painful, swollen joints appear along with a return of fever. Antibodies that have been forming in response to the infection are attacking the connective tissue around arteries in the joints, and worse, in the heart muscle and valves. The fibrous tissue, particularly of the left-sided valves (mitral and aortic) degenerates and forms wartlike lesions on the valve leaflets, a process that greatly interferes with heart function. Fortunately, rheumatic fever is rare in this country since the 1960s, but is still prevalent in much of the world. Also fortunately, it doesn't strike until its victims are older than five years of age. Much of the decline in cases is attributed to actively recognizing and treating group A infections. One other evidence of good fortune is that the organism is still susceptible to penicillin—the most effective and least expensive antibiotic.

Because of these devastating diseases, I feel this is one illness that should always be brought to a physician's attention. Besides the clinical signs that point to the diagnosis, a quick, definitive strep test is available. If the test is positive antibiotic treatment is begun, which gives dramatic results and negates the possibility of these serious complications.

I saw lots of rheumatic fever and its devastating effect on the heart valves in medical school and residency training. Penicillin was and still is the antibiotic of choice unless a local hospital laboratory has found resistant strains of strep. Before the strep tests were developed, observing clinical signs, followed by penicillin therapy, markedly cut into the incidence of rheumatic fever. I have not seen rheumatic fever and only one case of glomrulonephritis (not my patient) in my practice. I am certain that the judicious use of antibiotics—used only when needed—is a factor that contributes to their effectiveness and prevents the development of antibiotic resistance. It is amazing that the original antibiotic, penicillin, is still the first-line antibiotic for this illness.

Few infants with a strep infection exhibit these signs of infection; a toddler, more. In this age group, then, rely more on whether the little one is "sick" and leave the diagnosis to your doctor. You'll have a strong head start for arriving at a diagnosis if other family members have symptoms of strep.

Laryngitis

Laryngitis, nearly always caused by a virus infection, is easy to diagnose due to the hoarseness and barklike cough associated with it. Its infectious nature is noted by the way that it spreads among close contacts. On the other hand, bouts of spasmodic laryngitis seem to come out of blue in a seemingly healthy child. Until it is dealt with a few times, it might be a frightening experience, which can exacerbate the problem. An allergic basis is sometimes implicated, which makes sense since postnasal drip, caused by food allergy or infection, contributes to the laryngospasm. Look for the possible triggers and keep calm during a bout. Vitamin C is the best "medicine."

Bronchiolitis

Bronchiolitis is a disease that occurs in the first two years of life. Over half of cases are due to respiratory syncytial virus (RSV) infection, but the other viruses mentioned above can be causative agents. RSV epidemics occur annually. In adults, RSV infection often manifests as a nasty sinus infection or a cold of moderate intensity. Maternal antibody protection is weak but provides some protection for the newborn. The infant becomes very susceptible a short time later. We hope infants can escape exposure during their first year. Infection in subsequent years is not likely to cause serious disease, as there appears to be some carryover immune response that developed from even a mild earlier infection. Bronchioles are the terminal, smaller branches of the bronchial tree of the lung. Their pathways (lumens) are small and easily plugged by secretions and debris from infection. This makes it hard for air to pass in either inspiration or expiration. Inspiratory effort allows some air to get through, more than expiratory effort can push it back out, creating air trapped in the lungs (easy to detect by examination and x-ray). The infant exhibits shallow, rapid respiration as it attempts to stay ahead of the game. Since carbon dioxide is not being exhaled efficiently, blood chemistries are thrown out of whack. This situation may not improve for as long as three days, but often resolves within twenty-four hours.

Treatment

Feeding the infant with bronchiolitis is difficult, but fluids are needed. Intravenous (IV) fluids may be necessary with more severe dehydration or when the blood chemistries may need correction. The semi-reclining infant is placed in a croup tent in which humidified oxygen can be administered. The bronchioles have no ring of smooth muscle around them like the larger bronchi, so it is questionable whether adrenaline, as used to relieve asthma, will help. However, larger bronchi, which are responsive to adrenaline, are probably somewhat involved in the disease process. Less controversial is the use of corticosteroids, the powerful anti-inflammatory agents. Every little bit helps. Frankly, both physicians and parents are willing to try anything that is safe and could possibly help as they watch an infant struggle for every breath. All are grateful to see the return of more normal breathing.

Adenovirus Infection

This is a particularly nasty virus when infants are affected. An infection from one of the strains of adenovirus may start out as a simple cold, but soon is seen to produce the most troublesome gunk (there is no better word) in the nasopharynx. This material irritates and inflames the surrounding tissues, causing the infant to easily gag and choke if it is allowed to pool in the back of the throat. The infant will be more comfortable, and safer, if put in a semi-reclining position while in this state. Lightly swaddling the arms should be calming. If not, put the infant or child on his or her side without restricting arm movement. (See the SIDS section and consider "tummy" position.) When putting the infant down for sleep, clear the nose, as with a head cold, as much as possible.

The striking amount of inflammation in the nasopharynx creates a strong potential for secondary middle ear infection—best prevented by clearing the area with the bulb syringe and saline drops, and with extra vitamin C. But if there is increasing fussiness and/or a return of fever, the possibility of middle ear infection should be checked, professionally, along with other considerations.

SUMMARY

Bad viruses are always lurking in the shadows. Some infants will have several colds before their first birthdays. Others will have none, even though exposure rates were similar in the two groups. The reason lies in the health of the infant's immune system and, in the immediate newborn stage, the immune health of mother. Whether or not an infant has inherited "good" or "bad" genes, even the "bad" can be strengthened to do a more favorable job through proper diet and added vitamin supplements. And parents can greatly help their child get over the acute infection when they know the expected course of these respiratory infections and utilize the almost mechanical, physical treatment methods we have suggested. Regular supplemental vitamin C goes a long way to achieving prevention, and helping to quicken cure.

Hygienic measures are important in reducing infection rate. An infected person should be careful not to send droplets of nasal secretions (with infectious viruses riding piggyback) into the air or onto hands. Of course, an infant does not respond to this suggestion, so the caretaker must do everything possible to stay out of range and wash their hands more frequently. Fortunately infants don't develop a forceful cough. Many parents go overboard when considering the germ theory of disease, with compulsive use of antiseptic wipes for hands and such things as banisters. During illness, dodging droplets is best. But for prevention, both short-term and long-term, rewards are greatest by achieving good immune health.

CHAPTER 9

FEVER: ITS SIGNIFICANCE AND MANAGEMENT

Fever is often not considered as just part of an illness but has a significance all its own. I have had mothers say, "My baby has a *temperature*." I refrain from answering, "I'm glad to know that" until I can explain that fever is a body temperature higher than normal, but is not altogether bad. Body temperature will increase in a warm-blooded animal whenever heat is not allowed to escape from the skin or the cooling effect of evaporating sweat is thwarted—this mechanism enables us to counter high ambient temperatures, as in the desert or the interior of a car parked in the sun. Fever due to infection is part of our body's method of stimulating the immune system to counter the invasion of bacteria or viruses. I emphasize that fever is part of an illness but not the illness itself. What needs to be determined is whether or not the child with fever is "sick." Evaluate after successfully getting the fever down. If sick, see the doctor without worry of not being specific—especially in the case of an infant—don't engage in self-diagnosis. If not sick, withhold treatment of any kind for a moderate fever, unless the child is uncomfortable at bedtime. Even then, use fever medicines sparingly—I will explain the pitfalls of fever drugs (including Reye's syndrome). Fever gets the immune system in gear. It has a purpose.

FEVER: ITS DESCRIPTION AND MANAGEMENT

At the onset of infection, there might be chilling. Actual shivering with muscle contractions generates heat, like lighting the burners in a boiler.

The infant should be bundled up and carefully observed until any goose bumps are gone and the skin of the trunk is warm to the touch. Then allow heat to dissipate more readily from the body with light clothing and bedding.

The essential thing for an infant, more so than with an older child who can tell you what hurts, is to evaluate the sickness that is causing the fever. How does he or she look? Is he listless or terribly irritable, less social than usual, with an unwillingness to make eye contact, pale—in other words, *sick?* If temperature has risen rapidly, to the point of making the infant jumpy, not only is evaluation of the underlying illness difficult, but it is time to work on lowering the fever. A more meaningful evaluation of the illness can be made once that is successful.

Mothers usually need no precise instruction to tell them when their baby is sick. Criteria for evaluating illness based on set elevations of fever should not usurp this instinctive insight. Infants don't always follow the norm suggested by the experts. Infants should be evaluated whenever parents have feelings of dread from what *they* feel is a sick infant. When a mother from the barrio would call in the night and say, "My baby *seek*", I knew I had to see them, regardless of the time of night. Infections in infants progress so much more rapidly than in older children that professional evaluation should be considered whenever "home diagnosis" seems shaky.

Treatment of Fever—And When to Do It

When an infant becomes irritable, jittery, and hot, all at the same time, heat is not leaving the lightly clothed body fast enough. The fever does its job at temperatures below what brings on these signs and symptoms, so it has now become a nuisance. It is time to treat. I have not seen febrile seizures (convulsions associated with fever) in infants, but I have experienced this disturbing and frightening event in toddlers. Though not common, a seizure is more likely to develop when the temperature rise is abrupt and achieves a high level (around 104°)—much like an exaggerated shaking chill. The little one should be put on his or her side or tummy so that anything in the mouth will not interfere with breathing. It will seem to last an eternity, but I have not witnessed a duration of over two minutes, even though they can last up to fifteen minutes and still be included in this less serious category. Maybe fifteen minutes of convulsing is not considered "serious" to a statistics gatherer, but it sure is to parents or doctors who witness the event. I am sure the duration is shorter if the first-line cooling method of cool sponging is employed. A febrile convulsion does not cause brain damage.

Sponging is very effective if it is started as soon as hot skin is detected. Expose the skin of the trunk, which is the most accessible and the most extensive area. If she doesn't mind being on her tummy, place her on an open diaper. Adding the skin surface of the buttocks and the backs of the upper legs greatly aids the effectiveness of sponging. Place a bowl of tepid water—not too warm; not too cold—by the crib-side. Use a cloth large enough to cover all the exposed skin. Wring it out in the water, and spread it over the entire exposed skin. The cloth should be of thin enough material that you can feel the heat in the cloth as it is transferred from the skin. By soaking the cloth, wringing it out, and reapplying, noticeable cooling will take place after just a few cycles. This method transfers body heat into the bowl of water. The trick is to find the right temperature of the water to start with. We have heard of alcohol sponging utilized in hospitals for adults. Babies don't say, "Yikes!" but they certainly can cry in protest. Evaporation of alcohol from an infant's skin creates discomfort and would never be effective, since the surface blood vessels would immediately shut down and the blood would go to the interior of the body for warming. If the sponging water is too cold, the same thing happens. The right temperature will not be uncomfortable and it will be effective.

During fever there is considerable water loss from the body. Every hot breath is loaded with water vapor. Infants are especially intolerant of dehydration. Appetite is depressed at a time when calories are being burned to increase body heat. Clear liquids, in small amounts, need to be offered often. Breast-feeding should go according to need—the infant will only take what is needed at the time, with water in between. Avoid overfeeding of the bottle-fed infant. Lower caloric intake for the few days of the illness will have no long term effects, but paying attention to fluid intake is a must. One of the over-the counter pediatric electrolyte preparations may be considered if fever persists and the infant is off his feed and liquid intake.

Medication

I never prescribed fever-lowering, pain-relieving medications for infants less then three months of age. The heat-dissipating measures usually sufficed. I later raised the age threshold to six months, below which I did not prescribe. I did not want to mask any signs of the causative illness, such as irritability or the fever itself. I prescribed low, weight-appropriate amounts of aspirin. Baby aspirin was a 1.25 grain (81 milligram) preparation. For three to six months, just one-half a grain (or roughly half of a baby aspirin) and little more for the six months to one year age group. A two-and-a-half-year-old would be given two baby aspirin. These doses should not be given more than four times in twenty-four hours, and were not to be given once the temperature was down to a comfortable level. The best use of aspirin was for comfort at bedtime, so that the infant (and parents) might have a restorative night's sleep. I have chosen the past tense, because, currently, aspirin for infants is frowned upon. Later on we describe the thought that conservative use caused no trouble. But why give anything if it isn't needed?

Reye's Syndrome

Reye's syndrome is a terrible disorder in which a previously healthy child rapidly becomes desperately ill from liver failure and encephalopathy. I saw my only case of Reye's syndrome when in consultation for another doctor. Both of us were haunted by the outcome. This twelve-year-old boy was in the last throes of the disorder. He was hospitalized with uncontrollable vomiting and mental confusion during an influenza epidemic. His liver was greatly enlarged. He had to be restrained to avoid injury from his wild thrashing and crying out. Fortuitously, I had just read an article that very morning, in the medical journal *Pediatrics* about this newly recognized syndrome. This was in 1963. The article dealt with the syndrome that doctors had described in the British medical journal *Lancet*. The authors suggested that aspirin administered to children during the course of a viral disease, especially chicken pox and influenza, could induce liver malfunction leading to high blood ammonia levels, low blood sugar levels, and brain degeneration and swelling (encephalopathy). We had a diagnostic label but no idea how to help this child. By 1987 it was found that some survivors of the syndrome had various metabolic disorders. The authors concluded that there were predisposing conditions that would lead these children to developing the syndrome.[1] If caught early, we now know that there are heroic efforts that can save many.

Our CDC and FDA quickly and decisively condemned the use of aspirin in children (at one time all under nineteen years of age) during influenza-like illnesses or chicken pox. Aspirin (acetylsalicylic acid) is a salicylate. Salicylates are added to many processed foods and were curtailed during this period of clamp down, notwithstanding the fact that they occur naturally in many foods. Parents still are admonished to not use aspirin when a child has an influenza or chicken pox infection. But for general use, it can be used in a child over two years of age. I always suspected that I did not have any cases of Reye's syndrome in my practice because of my discussions with parents about the *minimal* use of aspirin, backed by a written instruction sheet. This idea was bolstered by an article in the *Journal of the American Medical Association,* which related doses of aspirin that were too high and too frequent to cases of Reye's syndrome.[2]

Acetaminophen, Ibuprofen, and Aspirin Safety

After recognizing the syndrome, Tylenol nearly completely replaced aspirin for use in children. This is the trade name for acetaminophen in this country, which has similar fever-lowering and pain-reducing properties as aspirin. The pharmaceutical company that makes it successfully made Tylenol (not just *any* old generic acetaminophen which is chemically identical) into a household word with advertising like, "Hospitals prefer Tylenol." Aspirin has regained favor because of the many physicians who prescribe low-dose aspirin for clot prevention in adults. Interestingly enough, articles are beginning to appear that find Reye's syndrome in adults who have been on a long-term daily aspirin program.

Acetaminophen is not perfectly innocuous. There is only a five-fold difference between an effective dose and a toxic dose. Acknowledgement of this has been slow in coming but has recently led to lowering the recommended dosage on the product label. Acetaminophen is a part of so many over-the-counter medicines—cold remedies and sleep enhancers, for example—that there is a serious potential problem when patients take these medicines, with their hidden doses, along with regular acetaminophen. This is the leading cause of liver failure in the western world.[3] The majority of these cases stem from the fact that medicines are taken too lightly while ignoring the cumulative effect derived from mixing a toxic drug like acetaminophen, for example, in with an over-the-counter sleep remedy. These attractively advertised drugs can be obtained without professional consultation. In the December 1976 issue of *Pediatrics,* Joseph Little noted the similarity of acetaminophen liver toxicity and the liver pathology of Reye's syndrome.[4] The 1987 article in *Pediatrics* stated that even acetaminophen, the substitute for aspirin, could cause Reye's syndrome.[5]

After aspirin was essentially blacklisted and replaced with acetaminophen, ibuprofen became "the new kid on the block." Its most common trade names are Advil and Motrin. Along with aspirin and many other similar drugs, ibuprofen falls in the category of nonsteroidal anti-inflammatory drugs (NSAIDs). Ibuprofen is on the market in a form suitable for delivery to infants. It has had recommendations for using it by itself for fever control, or alternating it with acetaminophen. Which treatment form is better is still debated. Unlike the NSAIDs, acetaminophen relieves discomfort but does not relieve inflammation. The alternating protocol would only provide anti-inflammation properties once every eight hours.

Inflammation is a base cause of many diseases; so NSAIDs have had wide use for treatment, or more often for symptomatic relief, of many chronic diseases. The biochemical basis for their action is faulty—the desire would be to stop production of the "bad" substance (a prostaglandin) that creates inflammation, while preserving the production of anti-inflammatory substances (other prostaglandins). These drugs seem to work well for short-term use. Long-term, not so well; problems are emerging in adults with such things as an increase in "cardiac events" due to suppression of "good" prostaglandin production. One by one these drugs have come under scrutiny. A few have earned a "black warning label" on the package insert to warn doctors who prescribe. But most have an over-the-counter (OTC) status that detours around physician advice.

Aspirin seems to be invulnerable to attack, thus far. There are far too many adults taking aspirin for another function, shared in part with all NSAIDs: preventing the clumping of blood platelets and subsequent clot formation in unhealthy arteries. Aspirin's action lasts for the lifespan of the platelet, while the other drugs have a shorter duration of action. Originally this practice was intended for those who had experienced a coronary event, but it morphed into a preventive measure in an attempt to spare people from heart attacks. A closer look is being taken concerning the wisdom of this approach with the recent discovery of problems with long-term use. There is a lot of pressure applied by the makers of aspirin to keep their good thing going.

SUMMARY

As with so many things, knowledge can dispel worry. Moderate fever is not a disease in itself but a natural response of our infant's body when it is being invaded, most commonly, by bacteria or viruses. Inflammation from other causes may produce fever in a toddler or older child. Whatever the cause, fever aids resolution and should be considered helpful.

As we learn the pitfalls of pharmaceutical treatment of fever in adults and the value of moderate fever in combating infectious diseases, why would we thoughtlessly use these drugs for treating infants? Sure, judicious use may be worthwhile when heat dissipation methods are not adequate. It all points to a simple medical philosophy: don't put something foreign into a body, especially a child's (or worse, an infant's) unless there is a clear benefit to risk ratio. The package insert provided with many prescribed drugs state that they are not to be used in infants because there have been inadequate safety studies. This precaution may or may not be heeded, and it certainly cannot be heeded in OTC drugs. I also tell my adult friends to consider the flip side of these warnings: If a drug is not safe for infants, is it *completely* safe for you?

CHAPTER 10

ALLERGIES

We put allergy problems in infants and toddlers into groups, defined by signs and symptoms we can observe: gastrointestinal, upper respiratory (nose and throat), lower respiratory (coughing or asthma), and skin.

The basis of an allergic reaction is an immunological response, much the same as with vaccinations. An antigen (allergen) stimulates antibody production that will keep this foreign protein invading the body under control. In considering bacterial invasion we can appreciate that, basically, this is a protective mechanism. The first exposure to an antigen is not noticeable. Antibodies are built in response to the specific antigen as a result of that first exposure. These antibodies have "memory" of the antigen and may quickly form antigen-antibody complexes upon subsequent exposure. There are two pathways that this reaction can take (these are described later). With allergy problems, the symptoms are not from the immune reaction itself, but from its side effects—the release of histamine and proinflammatory products that produce the signs and symptoms of the upset gut, the runny nose, and so on.

Our little ones have not had repeated exposure to most of the allergens that effect big people—those that would cause an antigen-antibody reaction. They pass through their first ragweed seasons with impunity. The potential allergens for them are mostly food allergens. For this reason, an upset stomach or intestinal tract would cast suspicion on food allergy, but the antigen-antibody complex can travel through the bloodstream and take up residence in the respiratory tree just as well. For decades, allergists had an incomplete concept of food allergy since it didn't fit the pattern of pollen and other sensitivities. The more comfortable term used was "food intolerance," which described symptoms but offered no explanation of its cause.

TYPES OF ALLERGIES

Before I (RKC) understood much about the immunology of allergy problems, I put what I saw in children into two basic types: (1) rip-snortin': including sneezing, wheezing, vomiting and intestinal cramping, hives, or, rarely, the worst possible reaction, called angioneurotic edema or anaphylaxis. The allergen enters the body through the respiratory tree, through ingestion, or more directly into the bloodstream through the administration of a shot. (2) Milder food allergies: what Dr. William Cook, a pediatric allergist, called "hidden food allergies." I would put an itchy, runny nose (clear mucus), mild intestinal cramping with mucus in the stools, or a long-lasting rattling cough (caused by post nasal drip) into this second group. Both kinds of allergy problems are categorized according to the organ system(s) they affect. Food allergies can manifest in about every system, including combined systems. Angioneurotic edema has its dangerous effect spread from the bloodstream to affect all systems. The alarming, life-threatening signs of laryngeal edema—hoarseness, then choking, and being unable to get a good breath—certainly get our attention. In this case immediate help is needed in the form of an injection of adrenaline.

Prostaglandins

Prostaglandins are similar to the hormones produced by groups of cells (as in the pancreas or thyroid) except they reside in cell membranes, ready to go to work (for good or bad) when stimulated to do so. The omega-3 fatty acids (mainly derived from oily, cold water fish) contribute to the formation of what we might call "good" prostaglandins, those that prevent inflammatory reactions in the body. The omega-6 fatty acids (derived from grains) form arachidonic acid, which produces proinflammatory substances and might be called "bad" prostaglandins.

The influence of these two kinds of fatty acids is not direct, but they affect the type of prostaglandin formed in the body. These, in turn, determine the type of antibodies that will be formed, type 1 helper (Th1) cells or type 2 helper (Th2) cells. The "bad" prostaglandin, PGE2, goes the Th2 route. Th2 antibodies lead to allergy antibodies called IgE. Th2 antibodies are humoral (in the bloodstream) and are formed during pregnancy. Th1 antibodies are tissue antibodies. The newborn needs to shift to the production of Th1 antibodies for their immune protection from many infectious agents now that the protection of the mother's antibodies has been removed. After birth, exposure to certain bacterial infectious agents will have a strong influence on encouraging the shift. The bacterium that causes whooping cough (pertussis) is one of these agents.

The Concept of Allergy

For decades, pediatric allergists held to the concept that "food allergy" is not allergy at all unless certain criteria are met—criteria similar to those accepted allergies I call rip-snortin'—such as positive blood tests for IgE gamma globulin, positive skin scratch tests or prick tests, and being responsive to desensitizing therapy. Fortunately, in the last few years, more and more doctors are accepting the idea that the shift away from the Th2 to the Th1 pathway will reduce the increasing incidence of infant and childhood allergy problems. The upshot of this is that they are taking a hard look at the newborn's environment. Has it been too sterile? Are we weakening or preventing the necessary shift? Also, more thought is being given to the role of omega-3 fatty acids in the immune system and how the balance of omega-6s and omega-3s affects it. One dramatic change is that some are entertaining the concept of desensitizing children with peanut allergy (under close observation in the doctor's office) with increasing homeopathic doses of peanut antigen. Perhaps, one day we "peanut terrorists" will be able to enjoy an in-flight peanut snack again.

The gamma globulin IgE is correlated with "stronger" allergies and used to be considered *the* blood test to determine the diagnosis of allergy. Fortunately, with advances of immunology, more consideration is being given to the lesser allergic reactions that produce an antibody in the gamma globulin G (IgG) class. An IgG antibody is the antibody found in the blood for a past infection (as opposed to a current infection). Now it is accepted that allergens can also produce this type of antibody response, which sort of legitimizes the term, "allergy." Since both the infection and the allergic response produce inflammation, we can see an overlap of allergy problems and infectious diseases, both in symptoms and treatment.

Pets: The More, the Better. Really.

An article appearing in *The Journal of the American Medical Association* entitled "Exposure to Dogs and Cats in the First Year of Life and Risk of Allergic Sensitization at 6 to 7 Years of Age" offers evidence that thinking is beginning to change regarding allergies in children and how best to avoid them.

According to this study, "Childhood asthma is strongly associated with allergic sensitization. Studies have suggested that animal exposure during infancy reduces subsequent allergic sensitization. . . . Of 835 children initially in the study at birth, 474 (57 percent) completed follow-up evaluations at age six to seven years. . . . The prevalence of any skin prick test positivity (atopy) at age six to seven years was 33.6 percent with no dog or cat exposure in the first year of life, 34.3 percent with exposure to one dog or cat, and 15.4 percent with exposure to two or more dogs or cats." The authors conclude, "Exposure to two or more dogs or cats in the first year of life may reduce subsequent risk of allergic sensitization to multiple allergens during childhood."[1]

This well-conducted study is one of confirmation of our having been overprotective in the way we attempt to prevent allergy problems developing in our youngsters. Our definition of "etopy" includes the more severe allergic reactions such as asthma and eczema. We describe the immunology pathway that gives the physician clear evidence of the allergen, based on blood tests and skin-prick tests. Allergists stuck with this paradigm for fifty years, many saying, "If the condition does not meet these criteria, it isn't allergy."

For decades, generalists and pediatricians advised that their little patients avoid early exposure to the potent allergens, like animal dander and some foods. We were admonished to delay offering foods, such as eggs (egg white is the culprit), fresh fruit (including orange juice), and fish until at least six months of age. Less potent, but common foods, like wheat, were also not to be given early. The only acceptable juice was apple. I would not completely discard this practice. I still advise cautious introduction of all foods, due to individual differences in the way the immune system responds and to avoid the less severe, but nevertheless annoying, allergy disorders.

Since cow's milk usually produced a milder form of reaction, infant formulas were usually acceptable, but breast-feeding was encouraged to continue at least for six months—this was a good spin-off. Studies showed that this worked *during infancy*. But we needed studies like this animal dander study to show us that this protocol did not bode well for the child.

Hair of the Dog, Cat, or What-Have-You Is a Good Thing

Only in the last few years are we told of studies like this that suggest we have taken the wrong pathway in trying to avoid allergies. Rather than avoid antigen exposure in the early months, we should encourage it. As conscientious (or compulsive) as we might be, we should abandon the concept of a sterile environment for our babies and be more down to earth. Farm-raised kids are doing better, allergywise, than their city-raised counterparts. It was suggested, in this study, that there are usually more farm-raised kids in a family than in city-raised families—greatly enhancing the spread of "germs," and putting their immune systems on the right track.

Gastrointestinal Allergy

We start with gastrointestinal (GI) allergy because it would be the first type of allergy to appear in an infant. (GI allergy was referred to both in the colic and the infant feeding chapters of this book.) Our newborn got along fine in his or her mother's womb. Then the only feedings were milk (breast or formula) for some time. Environmental exposures (inhalants, animal dander, molds, or dust) haven't been in the baby's environment long enough to cause an immune response.

Consequently, we have pretty much narrowed down the culprit to cow's milk. In itself, this makes a good argument for introducing foods later and cautiously, avoiding common allergens like wheat, eggs, and orange juice. When possible, nursing exclusively until the baby is six months of age is best. However, now we are faced with the new paradigm described above. I conclude that avoidance can be overdone, but, still, I would not advise introducing those foods that have the potential for the development of severe allergic reactions before six to nine months of age.

Cow's Milk Allergy

An allergy to cow's milk can start with a bang in an infant. Not just spitting up, but actual forceful vomiting (projectile vomiting) can be a consequence. An infant has little tolerance for repeated vomiting. This condition warrants a doctor visit to rule out pyloric stenosis, an obstruction at the end of the stomach. A skilled examiner can feel the enlarged muscle that regulates how long foodstuff remains in the stomach before it passes into the small intestine. Although it is very disturbing for a new mother to contemplate surgery for her infant, a pediatric surgeon easily (as far as *the doctor* is concerned) slits the muscle and loosens the grip, which provides almost instant relief. If this condition is ruled out, cow's milk allergy is considered.

Once it is confirmed that keeping water down is not a problem, an infant with a cow's milk allergy is put on a hydrolyzed protein, hypoallergenic, formula. Rarely, milk allergy occurs in a breast-fed infant. Whole molecules of milk protein can sneak from mother's intestinal tract into her bloodstream—and from there into her breast milk. I suspect that milk allergy may cause pyloric stenosis itself, through a similar mechanism. This can't be proven, because no time can be allowed to observe relief from the hypoallergenic formula. Often, a soybean-based formula is substituted before going to the hydrolyzed protein formula (which smells and probably tastes like wallpaper paste). This too can become an allergen in time, and will necessitate moving on to the broken-up cow's milk casein protein formula. The surprising thing is that either the soy formula or the hydrolyzed protein formula—so foreign tasting to us when compared to the nice tasting formula—is immediately accepted and "chowed down" by the infant.

Food Allergy

Food allergy is a common cause of intestinal upset. Allergy becomes the number one suspect if infectious diarrhea, viral or bacterial, or diarrhea following an antibiotic's effect of upsetting the intestinal flora is ruled out. Messy diapers are more frequent with a food allergy, but they don't have the "sick" odor of infectious diarrhea. In more severe cases, there will be cramping noted by distention of the abdomen and clear mucus in the stool. If this is even more severe there may be blood in the stool. This blood, which is from further upstream in the baby's gastrointestinal tract, is dark and can contribute a characteristic odor to the bowel movement. The appearance of blood gets the immediate attention it deserves and leads to the hypoallergenic diet.

The toddler, as we are all aware, is different. His milk allergy can be expressed as constipation. Maybe not so different, once one considers that an adult with "irritable bowel syndrome" can suffer from either diarrhea or constipation. There often is a perianal rash that itches, as if the milk protein acts like a contact allergen.

The detective work necessary when searching for the cause of an allergy problem is easier with an infant than a toddler, as there has been less time for multiple exposures to allergens. This is particularly true when searching for a food allergen.

Symptomwise, differentiating wheat allergy (allergy to the protein, gluten, contained in several grains) from what is called gluten sensitivity is difficult. Celiac disease, the serious auto-immune disease manifestation of gluten sensitivity, in which intestinal lining cells are destroyed, is very rare in infants or toddlers and deserves little space in this book. I mention it because gluten sensitivity is becoming a top health topic. A gluten-free foods industry is developing. Supermarkets have sections of gluten-free foods (not always as advertised). It is almost like a badge of honor to have gluten sensitivity, based on self-diagnosis. Medical practitioners should encourage their patients to pin down an accurate diagnosis by the elimination and challenge method.

This is the most reliable method (even better than allergy blood or skin tests) for pinning down a food allergen.

1. **Culprits:** Get some "suspects" in mind. Consider the common allergens, such as cow's milk, wheat, egg, orange—on through the "exotics"—chocolate, strawberries, and so on. Firm up your suspicions by keeping a food diary. When the allergy signs you are trying to eliminate are produced in relationship to food or drink intake, write down *everything* ingested. This list would detail every ingredient of, say, spaghetti. With nasal allergy, an itchy palate might come on almost immediately. There is often a longer interval between ingestion and obvious signs with a GI allergy or asthma, so go back several meals. "Fast" reactors, therefore, are easier to detect. Act on your findings by going on to the next step.

2. **Elimination:** Stop offering the suspect foods and allow three to five days to get them out of the system. You have hit the jackpot if the signs and symptoms disappear, and you can move to step 3. If not, keep searching.

3. **Challenge:** If symptoms return when you add the suspected offender back into the diet, this will provide all the proof you need. Stay away from that food or drink for a few weeks. Periodically, if the child is doing well, a "rechallenge" may be in order. The nice thing about the "allergy load" concept is that although every mild allergen was not detected, getting rid of some stronger ones prevented the additive effect that was sufficient to cause allergy signs and symptoms.

Nasal Allergy

Symptoms of nasal allergy can become apparent at a very tender age. And, by far, cow's milk is the number one suspect. The condition seemed to flourish with the introduction of commercial infant formulas in the 1950s. Prior to these new formulas, evaporated milk with added carbohydrates was in vogue. I have wondered if the difference in allergy reactivity might be due to subjecting milk to high temperatures in the evaporated milk processing, which denatured the protein.

My pediatric training at Los Angeles Children's Hospital was blessed by the presence of Dr. Arthur Parmalee. He was nationally well respected for his pediatric health tips, written for several magazines. Obviously, he was in the evaporated milk camp when he stated, "I am getting allergic to all this talk of milk allergy." I had completed the whole loop of diagnosis and successful treatment of cow's milk allergy with my three-year-old daughter by then. The wonderful thing about a doctor like Dr. Parmalee was that he listened. He allowed me to conduct a special outpatient clinic for infants and children with runny noses, rattling coughs, or intestinal upsets—after other causes had been ruled out.

When the blood-borne antigen gets to the mucous membranes of the nose, stuffiness, excessive clear mucus, and even itching ensues. Itching is much more easily seen in the toddler, but the infant might rub its nose on mother's best dress while being burped or be seen rubbing its nose on the bedsheet.

A toddler with nasal allergy often gives the "allergic salute." Our noses have three tiers of turbinates projecting from the outside toward the septum in the middle. Their function is to warm and humidify incoming air. While looking in a mirror, tilt your head back a little and push up the tip of your nose. This will expose the lower turbinate. The allergic salute does this and increases the air space between the swollen turbinate and the nasal septum. It is usually followed by a noticeable sniff.

When there is copious mucus production, the baby can have a rattling cough as the mucus pools in the back of the throat, or sometimes it seems that the baby has a hard time getting out of the way of it all. This is one more reason for my dislike of the supine position of sleeping (see the SIDS section). In the toddler, noisy coughing described as akin to that of a trained seal, if it is originating from the larynx, or a "brassy" cough, if derived from deep down, may be due to either infectious agents (see common problems chapter) or allergy. An excessive amount of mucus in the wrong spot can create sounds that mimic a "cold," chronic bronchitis, or laryngitis (see the chapter on respiratory illnesses).

PHYSICIAN, HEAL THYSELF

Before I (RKC) was "hep" to some of the nutritional aids that I now understand, I was still bothered with nasal allergy—some foods and some inhalants. In med school, the combination of grass pollens and cat dander just about did me in. While operating in "cat lab," my nose leaked all over the operating field. The first house call I made, after my move in 1970, was to visit a prominent family to see a little guy with asthma. The exam was going along, in a professional manner, until my nose started running all over the place. As I was writing out my instruction sheet, I finally noticed a cat lying behind me on the top of the couch I was sitting on. This confirmed my tentative diagnosis, while causing me great embarrassment!

Lower Respiratory Allergies and Asthma

Sometimes in children in as early in life as the toddler age group, we can begin to differentiate the noises of "bronchitis." Is it just "rattling" in the throat, or does the noise emanate from deeper down? An adult can "cough up," gather the material, and spit it out. If the material chronically is clear mucus, this rules out an infectious basis. If it is consistently yellow or green, chronic infection is suspected (now frequently called chronic obstructive pulmonary disease, or COPD). The younger the patient, the more difficult it is to differentiate bronchitis caused by infection from asthma, because "all that wheezes is not asthma." Whether caused by infection or allergy, a wheeze is produced by bronchospasm—a narrowing of the sleeve of muscle surrounding the bronchi. Think of the noise produced by forcing a fluid (including air) through a narrowed tube such as a kinked hose, or by letting air out of a balloon while pinching off the stem. Now that is a *real* wheeze.

In infants, infection is the precipitating cause of wheezing, not allergens. This also holds true through the toddler age group. This may be called "reactive bronchitis," as it is inflammation that causes bronchospasm. Infants can respond to airborne precipitators of bronchospasm, whether they are strict allergens or just irritants. Tobacco smoke may be one or the other.

A toddler may be old enough to have become sensitized to animal dander or dust mites. If he or she shows any tendency to allergic disorders, keep the sleeping area free of animals and shaggy fabrics. Dust mites love shaggy rugs. The mite itself is not the culprit; its droppings are (they are nearly invisible but easily airborne). Keeping mites and dander to a minimum is a first priority. Vacuuming should always be done with the child out of the room. Rarely, we need to consider using mattress and pillow covers to keep mites at bay. Even if sensitivity grows stronger, detecting and eliminating other allergens—thus diminishing the "allergy load" and the necessity of desensitizing therapy, can minimize its effect.

Treatment

I don't recommend using anti-inflammatory drugs for infants; so avoidance is our one and only preventive tool. Exposures that bring about reactive bronchitis are sporadic.

Treatment for the infant and toddler is not nearly as straightforward as it is for the older child or adult. Aspirin, the most popular anti-inflammatory drug, is known to precipitate asthma attacks in many allergic individuals. And all drugs in this class have known undesirable side effects. The bronchodilating medicines used in older patients are very effective with allergy-based asthma, but are not as effective for reactive wheezing. The side effects of jitteriness or raising of blood pressure, used to individualize the dose, are difficult to measure in little ones. Bronchial secretions are thick and obstructive when there is wheezing. Water needs to be offered frequently between feedings to thin the secretions. High-dose vitamin C, which will tame the inflammatory response, is one of the few safe and effective modes of treatment. High dose vitamin C is essential if wheezing is caused by an allergic reaction, as vitamin C degrades histamine. Antihistamine medicines should be avoided, because they induce a counter-productive drying effect of bronchial secretions.

Nevertheless, if the infant is struggling with breathing, a careful evaluation followed by monitored treatment will be needed. An appropriate dose of adrenaline can be used in the doctor's office or hospital setting, and the response can be evaluated to see if an oral bronchodilator could then be helpful. When breathing is too labored, oral feedings may need to be replaced with intravenous (IV) fluids and hospitalization may be needed to provide oxygen delivery. One instance of hospitalization provides strong incentive to search for means of nipping an attack in the bud—at home. (See the respiratory infections section for more information.)

Skin Manifestations of Allergy

There are two types of allergy problems that affect the skin—contact dermatitis and blood-borne. Contact dermatitis develops from repeated application of a substance that has the potential of becoming an allergen. Most commonly, in the infant, it will occur in the diaper area, in which urine or bowel soiling breaks down natural skin protectors. The most common offenders are laundry detergents or an ingredient of a lotion or cream designed for soothing the skin in this area. Effective treatment is more prevention, derived from proactive detective work pinpointing the cause. Avoidance of the offender eliminates the specific cause but requires finding substitutes to improve skin health. For a diaper rash, hypoallergenic "waterproofing" ointments are used when exposure to the air is not an option. Until the rash clears, allowing time when the baby can just lie *on* the diaper, without being tightly pinned in, will hasten drying and healing of the skin.

The toddler also can become sensitized to allergenic substances that can create lesions on apparently normal skin. If the skin covered by shirts or undershirts is involved with slightly red, dry, scaly patches but the diaper area covered by with a disposable diaper is clear, then the laundry detergent or antistatic clothes dryer sheets are suspects. Topical medications are also suspects.

Here's a specific example: Advertising can lead one to believe that every break in the skin could lead to serious infection. Their answer lies in immediately applying an antibiotic ointment to the "owee"—specifically, an antibiotic ointment that can be purchased over-the-counter. Typically, one of its three ingredients is the antibiotic neomycin—great for killing bacteria by surface contact, but forbidden for systemic (internal) use due to kidney toxicity. The other two antibiotics also are strictly for topical use only. Originally, OTC Neosporin ointment was safe to use even in the eye, to treat conjunctivitis, since the ingredients and their concentrations in this big tube were identical to the by-prescription, expensive ophthalmic preparation. With more general use and misuse, some patients were seen to have a severe sensitivity reaction in the conjunctivae and surrounds, which—even though it was rare—was cause enough for me to discontinue using it for "pink eye." The new advertised Neosporin includes another known topical sensitizing agent, a topical anesthetic designed to make "owees" less bothersome. As with other contact allergens, the more times the sensitizing substance is used, the more likely it will become a problem. In this case, avoidance is the best "medicine." The idea that antibiotics should be used on a scrape or cut to prevent infection that might develop makes no sense. Indeed, it could lead to problems. The best triple-action preventive is still clean, dry, and appropriately bandage (if oozing).

Severe Reactions

The king of allergic reactions is termed angioneurotic edema or anaphylaxis. To break down the meaning of this medicalese, "angio" means blood vessels; "neurotic" refers to the nervous control over the muscular wall of arteries; and "edema" is fluid leaking from capillaries into the surrounding tissue. Anaphylaxis includes the same symptoms found in angioedema and can progress to total shock. Both conditions include hives and itching. I am not concerned about the proper use of terms, just their terrible consequences. I think of angioneurotic edema as usually caused by something ingested, and anaphylaxis from something injected that quickly gets into the bloodstream.

Angioneurotic edema may start with itching of the palate that rapidly progresses to swelling of the lips and around the larynx (as noted by the development of a muffled speaking voice and a cough that sounds like a seal's bark). There may be hives or just splotchy skin with some red areas and some pale areas. Signs of hoarseness should set off the alarm to quickly get medical help. A shot of adrenaline gives emergency relief, but there is only a very short time to react. If a toddler ever experiences angioneurotic edema, parents are prescribed an emergency kit containing a way to deliver adrenaline, to allow time, in a future attack, to get the child to emergency care. Then, a diligent search for the culprit must be undertaken. Until the mystery is solved the emergency pack must accompany the child whenever he or she is away from an emergency facility.

Anecdote: Anxious parents, who thought I might be able to help their son, brought a boy of around ten years of age to my office. He had twice received life-saving care (a perfect description) for angioneurotic edema in an emergency room setting. The key next step was to find the culprit antigen that was setting off these attacks, and that was what the parents expected from me—to be able to instruct them on the way to go about the detective work, and to convince them that this "far-out" idea could be true: that something ingested could cause such a severe reaction. The culprit proved to be a red dye in a breakfast cereal, which would not have been a suspect had they not carefully checked out *all* the ingredients in *everything* he ate.

SUMMARY

The best start for an infant is obtained from good maternal care, carried over to the nursing mother. This means a plant-based diet chock full of antioxidants, supplemented with vitamin C and vitamin E. Remember, with vitamin E, a little squirt from the capsule right onto a favorite served food is enough. Vitamin C will be discussed further in its own chapter. Get the baby on the right immune-function track with fish in her (mother's) diet or fish oil capsules. Breast-feeding is best, as it avoids common cow's milk sensitivity, but it is not essential. Either way, introduce new foods later (ideally, not until six months of age) and cautiously. New information pours in every day about the near-miraculous effects of high-dose vitamin D and its benefits for the immune system. But specific studies of an infant's optimal dose are lacking. At the same time, there are no reports of toxicity with much higher doses than were formerly recommended. I would say 800 international units (IU) is a good amount, but stay tuned.

These suggestions are relatively new. If they are put into practice on a large scale, I believe we will soon see a reversal in the current alarming increase of allergy among children.

CHAPTER 11

OVER-THE-COUNTER (OTC) DRUGS

"One grandmother is worth two M.D.s."
—ROBERT MENDELSSOHN, M.D., PROFESSOR OF PEDIATRICS

The profit-making potential for over-the counter (OTC) drugs is huge. Consequently, we are deluged with television and magazine advertisements. The concept of "truth in advertising" seems to have gone out the window. It has been replaced by a theme of "a drug for each and every symptom." A perfectly miserable-looking fellow in the "before" picture for the partaker of a "flu" remedy ad almost immediately looks greatly improved in the "after" picture. The real problem comes from applying this same attitude to young children and infants. Originally, if drugs were to be administered to infants, they always stood alone, never in combination with other drugs. Harmful drug side effects are very difficult to trace with combination drugs, especially in nonverbal infants. The purpose of this presentation is to point out the folly of most of these drugs, which are intended for use in adults or older children. By this, we can better understand the double folly of giving these drugs to infants. I checked the cold remedy shelves in a standard franchised drug store and went to the infant section. Admittedly, I began this project with a good deal of skepticism, since I had seen the demise of some useful products that were replaced with some that were not so useful. While on my knees, clipboard in hand, several people grabbed things off the shelves. I had to restrain myself from asking them, "Do you really want to buy that?" In spite of all the familiar trade names and attempts to convince the buyer of the specificity of action of *their* product, I found only eight ingredients, shuffled in various ways, to fill a large shelf of products. Mainly, just two antihistamines for allergy relief, one for cough suppression, one expectorant, two (mostly just one) decongestants and the standard two drugs for "pain and fever" relief.

BRAND-NAME OTC PRODUCTS

The colorful packaging is attractive and, along with the catchy names, a legitimate tool of marketing. There are products for such things as "stuffy nose and colds," "nighttime cough," "cough and cold," "allergies," or "multiple symptom cold medicine." Drug companies devise these clever names for their products based on symptom relief. I object to the use of a familiar household name, such as "Tylenol," for a product containing substances far removed from the acetaminophen that originally was the generic drug.

Benadryl

The brand name Benadryl was, and continues to be, well known. Although it is sold as an OTC product, alone or mixed with other drugs, doctors often recommended it as an antihistamine because of its safety record and the fact that it comes in a form that can be given as a quick-acting shot in the emergency room. Early on, the drowsiness side effect of this OTC product was noted, so it also became available as a nonprescription "sleeping pill." Worse, the pediatric liquid form, which had the yummy flavor of cinnamon, was abused by youngsters looking for a taste treat (with the help, of course, of an adult dispenser). Worse yet, a few preschool administrators were found to be keeping their little charges more compliant (and less likely to get into mischief) with Benadryl Elixir. Fortunately the Food and Drug Administration got wind of this practice and it became well publicized. This still widely used drug for adults now goes under its generic name, diphenhydramine, to avoid the bad reputation associated with the Benadryl name.

Dimetapp

You can also see many Dimetapp products on the shelf. Dimetapp was a popular antihistamine-decongestant combination in a tasty grape flavored elixir, allegedly *safe* for infants. The antihistamine was brompheniramine; the decongestant, phenylpropanolamine. Nothing like the original is available under the Dimetapp label now. The propanolamine was wisely replaced, first with psuedoepinephrine and then with phenylephrine, which creates less blood pressure response. The infant preparation substituted diphenhydramine, the old "Benadryl," for brompheniramine, but retained the latter in the adult product. All antihistamines carry a warning about the side effect of drowsiness. My personal experience tells me that brompheniramine (Dimetane) had the least of this side effect. (Adults can compare this with next best Chlortrimeton and Benadryl.)

Coricidin

One of the most egregious examples of marketing a new drug under an old, popular name is that of using the cover name Coricidin, which was the trade name for a simple combination of the antihistamine (Chlortrimeton) and a decongestant. Now we have a "cough and cold" Coricidin, consisting of dextromethorphan (DM) and chlorpheniramine; a combination acetaminophen and chlorpheniramine Coricidin; and the worst of the lot, Coricidin HBP (high blood pressure) for adults, which is a combination of the cough depressant dextromethorphan (DM), the expectorant guaifenesin, the antihistamine chlorpheniramine, and acetaminophen—the works—while omitting a decongestant that might cause a rise in blood pressure. ("Give me your fanciest hamburger, but hold the onions.") This product is unique only in that it omits the decongestant. The first-mentioned Coricidin above, along with Coricidin HPB, has become more popular as a means to achieve a "high" by overdosing—the products that contain DM. (If that is the desired effect, the purchaser better look at more than the Coricidin label and check the DM content.)

OTC MEDICATIONS FOR INFANTS AND YOUNG CHILDREN

Here is the lineup of OTC medications for children and infants (which are found on a special, separate shelf): For cough stoppers we have only one drug, dextromethorphan. For cough "loosener-uppers" (expectorant action) we have guaifenesin. The most popular antihistamine is diphenhydramine (Benadryl), followed by cetirizine (Zyrtec). I found only one product that used chlorpheniramine (Chlor-Timetron). In infant preparations, it can't be found alone but always combined with other drugs. My search also yielded no form of Chlor-Timetron for young children or infants, yet Chlor-Timetron syrup was widely used by pediatricians before it was combined with the other Coricidin products. The FDA is constantly demanding "black labels" (safety labels) for products such as these. So when a drug becomes unpopular, and it becomes unprofitable to manufacture, it is dropped from the market. Antihistamines are administered to counter the side effects of the histamine release, caused by allergic reactions. These lead to itching, sneezing, copious outpouring of mucus, swelling of mucous membranes, and, sometimes, wheezing. They are included in cold preparations in the questionable belief that inflammation from infection produces the same problems seen with histamine release. For decongestants in infant preparations, we now have only one—phenylephrine. A decongestant is designed to reduce the swelling in the nasal membranes to produce a freer airway. It does this through causing vasoconstriction in these tissues (see chapter 14 for information about the antihistamine effect of vitamin C).

There are just two drugs available to lower fever and relieve aches and pains in infant preparations: acetaminophen and ibuprofen. Ibuprofen is a nonsteroidal anti-inflammatory drug (NSAID)—certain steroids being the "granddaddy" of anti-inflammatory drugs. Aspirin also is a NSAID, but its use in children was condemned years ago when it was found to be associated with Reye's syndrome. Some children taking aspirin during an influenza or chicken pox infection developed this sometimes-lethal syndrome. (See the fever section for more information.) Acetaminophen is described below.

SIDE EFFECTS AND CHANGES IN FORMULATIONS

After phenylpropylnolamine was discontinued as a decongestant, it was replaced with pseudoephedrine (Sudafed). This drug is known to affect blood pressure, since it is prescribed for hypotension (when blood pressure is too low). Interestingly, it is also used as a psychotropic drug to boost the neurotransmitter norepinephrine. Unfortunately, Sudafed was being purchased in large quantities as an ingredient of homemade methamphetamine ("meth"). This led to regulation of sales and destroyed the good reputation of pseudoephedrine. We are now left only with phenylephrine—trade name Neo-Synephrine—used as a nose spray or drops as well as in oral preparations. One study states that it is ineffective compared to pseudoephedrine.[1] Big people can still find the stronger, longer-lasting and more bioavailable oxymetazoline (Afrin) nose spray, but it was deemed unsafe for infants. And later infant nose drops, containing even milder Neo-Synephrine, met the same fate.

Dextromethorphan, the alleged cough-stopper, is also used as a "recreational drug" in larger than recommended doses. Side effects for its use in infants include an increase in sudden infant death syndrome (SIDS), probably due to suppressing not only the cough but also respiration in general. One company uses it in its "daytime" product but omits it in its "nighttime" product, since nighttime breathing isn't tracked. In some products this gap is filled with diphenhydramine (Benadryl) to enhance sleep. There is no other cough suppressant approved for use in infants. Guaifenesin is the only approved expectorant. The two drugs often occur in the same preparation: "for coughs due to colds." There don't appear to be any side effects from guaifenesin, but when it is in combination with other drugs, side effects may be hard to spot.

Antihistamines, including diphenhydramine (Benadryl), produce a drying effect in the membranes of the nose and throat. As with any drug, there can be overdosing. As with all of these remedies, "polypharmacy" (effects from taking multiple drugs at the same time) must be considered.

Infants, particularly newborns (neonates), are not simply small versions of big people. Some drugs are known to create bizarre symptoms in neonates. A shocklike condition called "the gray baby syndrome" can arise from use of the antibiotic chloramphenicol. Benzyl alcohol is used as a preservative in IV fluids and is allegedly easily metabolized to harmless benzoic acid, *except* in neonates, where it can produce an alarming gasping, as if the baby is terminal. Its use in neonates was banned in the 1980s. Attempts to calm infants who were to undergo tests with phenobarbital backfired—it was much like giving catnip to a cat. For most cats, catnip acts like a "recreational drug." Other cats become hissing monsters, especially from too much. Rather than acting as a soporific (sleep inducer), phenobarbital proved to be a neuro-excitant for infants and young children.

Drugs need to be metabolized through enzymes produced by the liver to complete their intended assignments. An immature liver has not perfected this capacity. Some drugs are so foreign to the body that perfect metabolism will never be achieved. The cytochrome P450 enzyme is active in hormone synthesis and the breakdown of cholesterol and vitamin D, as well as toxic compounds including many drugs. Normal body metabolic processes compete with drugs for this enzyme. If there is not enough P450, a drug may not break down sufficiently and could rise to toxic levels. And drugs have intramural battles of their own when they enter the liver. Adults should be leery of an adult drug that has been determined unsafe for infants—that, to me, is a "canary in a coal mine."

Too much acetaminophen is a liver toxin. "Too much" is easy for a variety of reasons: (1) The directions on the bottle are willfully exceeded because of the attitude that "more is better." (2) Acetaminophen is a drug with one of the narrowest windows between an effective dose and a toxic dose. (3) Acetaminophen is often added in with other drugs into medications used for the discomfort of "flu and colds" or to reduce the discomfort that hinders sleep. The buyer isn't aware of the cumulative effect of taking different drugs for differing ailments simultaneously. One British study states that over half of the liver transplants in that country are due to acetaminophen toxicity—not from taking one big toxic dose, but from accumulating smaller doses.[2] Year after year, data from the American Association of Poison Control Centers indicates that acetaminophen is one of the most frequently reported drugs associated with unintentional poisoning. The FDA is trying to correct this problem with warnings and diminishing suggested doses on product labels. But old habits are slow to die—and how many study the label anyway?

Ibuprofen (one trade name being Motrin) in the NSAID class of drugs is subject to the same side-effect that plagues all of them—stomach bleeding—and should never be used long-term in any sized human being.

DR CAMPBELL'S OPEN LETTER TO PEDIATRICIANS

Since parents will more readily change the lifestyle of their child than of themselves, pediatricians get higher ratings for patient compliance to medical advice and education than internists. Parents leaving the pediatrician's office with a prescription should have full knowledge of what that medication can or can not do, or what it might do but shouldn't. Older pediatricians have seen the result of this kind of education passed on to the next generation.

Undermining our best efforts is the proliferation of over-the-counter drugs presented to the public in little short of a fraudulent fashion, that promotes a mentality of "if you have a symptom, any symptom, you owe it to yourself to wipe it out."

In a letter to the editor of *Pediatrics,* I wrote: "I was elated when I read the article 'Toxic Hydroperoxides in Intravenous Lipid Emulsions Used in Preterm Infants' in *Pediatrics,*[1] especially the discussion section that so clearly and completely explained the dynamics and harmful effects of free radical production from polyunsaturates.

"Those of us who give nutritional advice need this kind of information, which points to the necessary balance between iron, polyunsaturated fatty acids, antioxidants (particularly vitamin E) and the leukotrienes produced in cells in response to inflammation or trauma. Although the information was targeted for the neonatologist, it has a much broader application.

"My intellectual high crashed soon after, when I got a few pages further on in the journal: I ran across a two-page advertisement for five different over-the-counter products for 'Colds and Allergies,' 'Chest and Head Congestion,' 'Cough Relief,' 'Colds with Coughs,' and 'Maximum Strength Nighttime Relief for Children.' Expecting a precise description of the expected and known effects of the ingredients, I was disappointed to find the second page only showed a rogues gallery of a smiling patient, mother, and (most disappointing of all) a doctor, who had no business smiling after shirking his obligation to his patient. I searched for a listing of ingredients. Even scrutinizing the labels of the individual bottles with the aid of a powerful magnifying glass failed to reveal this information. In its stead was a deplorable laundry list of symptoms in lay terms: 'stuffy nose,' 'runny nose,' 'sneezing and itchy watery eyes,' 'chest congestion,' and 'quiets cough' (a hand over the mouth would accomplish the same thing). Not a word about the 'gunky' nose or 'tummy' ache that might result from all this symptom relief.

"Shouldn't the physician exercise a little discernment in order to help his patients wade through the muck of confusion produced by this advertising and labeling? Or should the patient just ask the pharmacist or the clerk, '"What's good for a stuffy nose?" Is the pharmacist really able, without any clinical history being offered, to discern whether the stuffy nose is due to nasal allergy or to strep nasopharyngitis? And neither the doctor nor the pharmacist can provide intelligent advice without reading the ingredients listed on the label.

"Unless the pharmaceutical companies list and describe ingredients, in an easy-to-read fashion, for these drugs, as they are required to do for prescription drugs, I feel strongly that the journal should drop their ads. Let us get back control over what our patients ingest."

Note: Perhaps this letter, addressed to the American Academy of Pediatrics, was well received, since some progress has been made. Ingredients now have to be listed, in print that is legible.

Reference

1. Helbock, H. J., P. A. Motchnik, B. N. Ames. "Toxic Hydroperoxides in Intravenous Lipid Emulsions Used in Preterm Infants." *Pediatrics* 91(1) (Jan 1993):83–87.

RATINGS AND SUBSTITUTES

The following is a list of OTC medications frequently offered to older children and adults and occasionally to infants and young children, and my evaluation of their efficacy and value. Always consider possible long-term consequences against any short-term benefits when treating your child with medication.

Phenylephrine (Sinus Congestion Relief)

Phenylephrine does not have a bad safety record. But as an oral product designed to cause vasoconstriction of the blood vessels of the nose, I wonder how a blood-borne drug could act so specifically and not affect blood vessels throughout the rest of the body. This is why I preferred the judicious use of nose drops—hit the enemy where it is and avoid collateral damage. But alas, infant nose drops are no longer available. This drug might be given my okay, but be aware of what it is combined with.

Dextromethorphan (Cough Relief)

Our infants do not require exposure to recreational drugs, especially so early in life. And here is the clincher—some studies have shown that it is not effective in children to suppress coughing (if so, surely not in infants). In the "Respiratory Problems" section, I have the remedy for coughing that is due, in infants, more to what is going on in the nose and throat than in the chest. Keep the nasal secretions cleared away and nose and throat membranes moistened through use of a humidifier. This drug rates the "forget it" classification.

Guaifenesin (Decongestant)

Although there are few reports of side effects caused by guaifenesin, one can hardly find a stand-alone expectorant. I find the best expectorant for children to be grapefruit or grapefruit juice. For infants, try to keep secretions thin with a good liquid intake and keep room air less drying with a humidifier. I would rate the drug as okay if one could find it unsullied by other drugs.

Antihistamines

All antihistamines have a drying effect, which is good if the child is sneezing great quantities of mucus (almost unheard of in an infant), but not good when the mucus automatically grows thicker as the cold progresses and further obstructs an infant's airway (which has a narrow opening to start with). I would challenge adults to do their own self-evaluation during the next cold I hope they don't get. I don't think the relief from OTC medications that contain an antihistamine are all they are cracked up to be. It substitutes a drippy nose with a dry throat—not good for infants. And the oral antihistamines in cold remedies are never alone. I hardly think that an infant minds having a runny nose. I prefer they have that rather than a discharge that is too thick to run. Replace antihistamine use with the same techniques as with decongestants. Rate: So-so. Possibly, but not necessary, for toddlers. "No" for infants.

Acetaminophen and Ibuprofen (Ache, Pain, and Fever Reducers)

It is very difficult to evaluate alleviation of aches and pains in infants or what to attribute apparent relief to. They cry from discomfort, and that is as specific a response as one can get. Their discomfort from a cold is more likely from not being able to breathe comfortably, and is alleviated by the means outlined above concerning decongestants. Ibuprofen's pain relief is also hard to evaluate. The fever-lowering ability of both drugs is iffy and is easily replaced with a "drugless" method outlined in the fever section of this book.

SUMMARY

At this point, I categorically say, *"Just say no to infant (OTC) drugs,"* not only because they are either harmful or ineffective, but mainly because more effective and safer means of relief can be found. There is no place for the drying effect of antihistamines, especially when one considers that high-dose vitamin C degrades histamine and is a true "anti" (more on this in the vitamin C chapter).

We will never know just what goes on in the infant brain, their perception of discomfort, or just what factors promote crying or sleeplessness. Therefore we should not attempt to apply "adult" solutions to problems we don't understand. We doubt if a low to moderate fever bothers a baby much. Crying is a nonspecific response to anything different. Always look for the cause, but crying may just be equivalent to an adult saying, "I feel lousy." With only the expression of fussiness as a means of communication, infants can't describe or exhibit either benefits or drawbacks to these drugs.

We "more articulate" big people should test these drugs on ourselves and make honest evaluations. While we extrapolate what we learn we should also remember that infants are more vulnerable to drug side effects, even after we adjust for weight. Drugs compete for the same enzyme systems in the liver to break down and be metabolized. This makes drug combinations problematic, especially for the immature liver of an infant. The livers of, in particular, the very young, the old, and many in between need all the help they can get to maintain their health, and this is best accomplished through good nutrition and vitamin supplements.

CHAPTER 12

CHILD REARING

*"Go see what your brother is doing
and tell him to stop it."*
—ATTRIBUTED TO SAM LEVENSON'S (1911–1980) MOTHER

I (RKC) don't want anyone to think of me as simple-minded. However, I admit to reducing "complicated problems" to simple explanations. Bullying, violent behavior, cheating, lying, disliking school, poor self-esteem, troubles from alcohol and/or drugs, can all stem from inadequate "bringing up" and modeling at home. There is a tendency to isolate each problem rather than thinking about the core cause. Headlines are full of examples of kids (and immature adults) who just don't seem to have a concept of right and wrong behavior, or how selfish acts affect others. Guidance has to start early. Very early.

WHO'S IN CHARGE?

An infant can get on the right track when Mom decides when and what her loved one eats. A feeding program must be entertained as soon as mother and infant leave the birthing place. A good place to start is always at the beginning. Develop a consistent pattern and there will be fewer problems later on. The older and smarter he or she gets, the more thought has to be given as to how to stay consistent and avoid what psychiatrists are calling the oppositional defiant disorder (ODD) (I choose to call this "bratting"). An intelligent toddler enjoys

169

the game of manipulating parents with their authoritarian ways. Remember, parents, you are bigger and wiser! *You* are in charge! There are numerous opportunities to show your love. Giving in to your little one's determination and defiant attitude isn't one of them.

Psychiatry has taken a dangerous path by attempting to make normal behavior a disorder or disease. Dr. James Dobson's book *The Strong-Willed Child*[1] explains how to deal with these dynamic toddlers without the parent also becoming defiant and creating a stalemate. Being obstinate is just a matter of the toddler not easily giving in in a match of wills. What is to be gained by tacking a diagnosis onto normal people, big or little? Nothing for the patient; a great deal for the doctor. When one of these obscure diagnoses makes it into the psychiatric diagnostic and statistical manual of psychiatric disorders (DSM), a listing of diagnoses with corresponding code numbers for the purpose of billing, then health insurance will pay for treatment and for establishing the diagnosis. Even adult grieving is being considered a treatable condition as if it represents abnormal behavior. Psychiatrists currently are saying that young children (close to the toddler age group) are being *under diagnosed* for bipolar disorder (formerly called manic-depressive disorder). At the same time they admit that symptoms are shared with oppositional defiant disorder and attention deficit hyperactivity disorder (ADHD)—two other nebulous disorders. Since one of the main purposes of diagnosing is to be able to bill for services (the other being the provision of a "scientific" reason for bad behavior that eliminates feelings of inadequacy for the parents), don't fall for this ploy. In the DSM-5, due to appear in 2013, the trend of calling normal behavior a "disorder" is increasing. A new entry will be "disruptive mood dysregulation" carefully defined as "children who exhibit persistent irritability and frequent episodes of behavior outbursts, three or more times a week for more than a year." What do you parents of a child in the "terrible twos" call these outbursts? How about temper tantrums? Perhaps we can work together and eliminate this behavior before the year requirement is up. Or maybe these outbursts will only occur *twice* a week and disqualify the child from acquiring an official psychiatric diagnosis.

Although there is equivocation as to just when it happens, there is a consensus of opinion that abstract thinking isn't very well developed until around age eight. "Reasoning" with a little one who is looking to stick scissors into an electric outlet is not appropriate adult behavior. Understanding behavior in the framework of a medical diagnosis is not possible with the toddler and it should not be necessary for the parent. Decide what is best for your child, enforce it with love (never anger), and be consistent. Boundaries of behavior will eventually become ingrained in this way, and then, later, understood. Very simple. Oh yes, good advice, but it requires a lot of determination to follow through. One word of comfort: It is the *smart* ones who are the most difficult to raise. Experienced parents and experienced educators (is there much of a difference?) can tell us how adults can turn these simple basics, which suffice for raising little ones, into complicated issues. No educator—whether parent or professor—can function effectively without sticking with the basics. It can be a rough job attempting to educate "students" who have not the foundation of acceptable behavior ingrained and practiced since early on in their education process.

Having taught every grade there is, literally from kindergarten to post-doctoral, my (AWS) experience confirms what Dr. C. states. Kids in school, at almost any age, know or quickly learn that the system is weakest at the top. If a child acts out, the teacher calls his or her name and gives the child more attention. If the child relentlessly misbehaves in class, that child is sent to the principal's office. If that does not work, then the child is put out of school and provided with a tutor. The take-home lesson? If you are bad, you get attention. If you are worse, you do not even have to sit in class. If you are really bad, you do not even have to attend school. This is learned behavior, and it starts powerfully early.

Adults reinforce bad behavior when they appease it. As one of my education professors said to me decades ago, "All kids learn in school, every day. The question is *what*." We might say that teachers are underpaid parents, but parents are utterly unpaid teachers. Before 8:00 A.M. or after 3:00 P.M., your kids are still students. *Your* students. Infants lock in on you and take in your every move. This literally begins at birth, and some of it is instinctual. In the animal kingdom it is called imprinting. Getting your ducks in a row may be hard for a hunter, but it is easy for a mother duck. They follow her from birth. However, she must be ever vigilant as to where she leads them. This goes for us male "mallards" as well. It soon becomes apparent that infants are individuals from the beginning. Some are more compliant; others continually make their presence known with their lungs and bodies in motion—minds always whirling. Parents of a "good" baby get more sleep at night than parents of an active, demanding baby. If the "hear me" baby begins to cry, it is best not to immediately run to the crib side. Let the crying go on long enough to see if it is designed just to solicit company or if it is calling for a problem fixer (a wet or dirty diaper, or genuine hunger). Of course intense crying calls for a look and comforting. Comforting (see the chapter on colic) can help differentiate real problems that might need medical attention from more readily controlled problems. It is not a good idea to immediately fill the "not as good" baby's request for motherly affection in the middle of the night, for fear of initiating a pattern.

Infants seem to have an innate sense that real needs will be met in answer to crying. Starting at a tender age, the less compliant infant will cry more often and with greater intensity. Over and beyond the relief of an immediate problem, there is the chance that crying can gain much more—companionship and the kind of comfort and loving kindness that is more appropriately given in the daytime, when all parties are fully conscious. Probably as soon as the second half of the first year, as awareness and consciousness increase, some infants begin to exercise their will. Parents have the difficult job of distinguishing the infant's *needs* from its *wants*, to avoid being overindulgent. And here is where the concept of "tough love" comes in. Just around the corner lurks the "terrible twos." If the parent falls short and gives in to a toddler's will, respect for authority is lost. To me, it is amazing that even a toddler can sense that: *When you really love me, you will make sure that I do the right things. I might enjoy the game of matching wills, but ultimately you're the boss.* By teaching in a loving way, you are also reinforcing respect, which will make the road easier in the next battle of the wills. Certainly, an infant, incapable of abstract reasoning, who is displaying annoying behavior, is not being defiant, but the remedy begins in infancy. There is nothing more exhausting than the task of instilling composure in a "wild" infant. In spite of fatigue and worrisome thoughts about how long this might continue, parents need to keep the good stuff in mind and know that, with love, they will end up with a delightful (but energetic) child. Fatigue multiplies negative feelings; so work out a plan that will assure needed rest. And give thought to the value of energy-building nutrition.

With an active but immature mind goes an active body. Accidents happen—spilled food, broken kitchenware, or worse—and can add up and make a mom's day tougher. But she recognizes that her precious toddler has not developed perfect coordination yet. Certainly, accidents should be separated from willful acts. The unchecked active mind and will can also lead to the defiance of authority that plays a part in eating patterns, bowel control, and sleep problems. (There is more on this in the chapter on infant feeding.)

Establishing Feeding Patterns

Feeding is more than getting the belly full, and the feeder can be neither too permissive nor too inflexible. We *offer*, not force feed, new foods. We want our love to be communicated to assist in the development of an attitude of loving good foods. The program may go nicely until the older infant learns the word "no," and exerts his or her will, and constantly tests parental authority. Then those in charge all say with one voice, *What do we do now? We don't dare let this precious little monkey win the battle of wills. We can't make him eat, and he can throw food at us. Should we let him starve to the point of crawling to us, begging for food?* I can't give a pat answer, my excuse being that individuals need individual treatment. This is why we do our best to retain the upper hand and not allow a dangerous pattern to develop. Repetition, with an early start, reinforces behavior. I know of one successful Stanford University graduate who put her parents through the wringer as a toddler. She subsisted on only peanut butter and a modicum of milk for months, even after her parents employed every known enticement that psychology could provide. The lesson is: Hang in there. (Peanut butter is a better brain food than celery, anyway.)

Pacifier Use

The "experts" seem to be forming a consensus that supports a new function of the pacifier as a sudden infant death syndrome (SIDS) preventer. I don't understand the rationale for this. Anything in the mouth promotes salivation, leading to material pooling in the throat and the potential for gagging and choking. (See the SIDS chapter.) A nursing mother who develops sore nipples from an infant who wants to constantly be on the breast *must* find an alternative. She is also admonished not to nurse lying down with the infant supine, because she might fall asleep and rollover onto her baby. Bottle-feeding should simulate natural breast-feeding as much as possible. I find a problem with a bottle-fed baby who is allowed to either feed from a propped up bottle while on his side or suck on a pacifier while placed on his back (as advised to prevent SIDS). It is difficult to determine sucking need. We don't often see a pacifier in a nursing baby's mouth in third-world countries where infants are exclusively breast-fed, often for two or three years. These babies are "demand-fed"—neither more often nor less often than in first-world countries—and seem to be content between feedings as long as the maternal supply is adequate.

I question how we evaluate "sucking need." The unborn, near-term baby makes sucking and swallowing motions, as if training for the big event (see Problems or Just Questions? Chapter]. Certainly, this does not continue all day or night long. Some infants seem to satisfy their sucking need each time they feed. If a breast-fed baby sucks frantically after nursing awhile, check with a breast pump to see what the actual volume of milk is in the feeding at the next feeding time. For a bottle-fed baby, check the mechanics of feeding—see if the nipple is too fast or too slow. If there is gulping while being bottle-fed, the nipple is releasing milk too quickly to be in tune with this vigorous feeder. The solution is to buy blind (unpierced) nipples, heat a needle red hot, and custom design the hole. Vigorous sucking sounds indicating poor flow would suggest enlarging the hole. If feedings go smoothly and the amount is adequate, but our poor, starving baby is still sucking like mad, perhaps pacifier use should be considered, during the daytime, until the baby is put down for sleep. Then remove it.

Why do I make such a big deal out of pacifier use? A lot of little deals add up to big deals. Good habits or bad habits have their beginnings early in life. Sometimes pacifiers are referred to as "plugs." Not a bad name when it is used to stifle crying in a less dangerous manner than by using duct tape. This is a particularly easy pattern to slip into. The very word "pacifier" implies a tranquilizing quality. When used in this way, we soon forget about "sucking need." If no thought is given to its use, a pacifier is automatically popped in whenever peace and quiet are desired. The longer this continues and the more hours of the day or night a pacifier is used, the greater the impact on the shape of the mouth and the dental arches. Commonly, one can see the effects of pacifier overuse in a child as young as three years of age. The result manifests as an overbite deformity (eventual buckteeth) and a shortened upper lip. The drawback I hate the most is seeing an obviously sharp twelve to fifteen-month-old making strange utterances in a frustrated attempt to get words out of a plugged mouth. There is no question in my mind that speech development is delayed with continuing pacifier use. When parents are *convinced* that it is time to do away with this habit, it is amazing how quickly even the most addicted infant can give it up. There is no patch for this addiction. Go cold turkey.

Some say pacifier use is the lesser of two evils, the other evil being thumb sucking. In rare situations thumb sucking can become so intense that the thumb becomes macerated and inflamed. In this case an attempt should be made to substitute the thumb with a pacifier, with time limitations.

Bowel Training

In considering bowel training and a matching of wills, the trainee *has it over the trainer.* So we must carefully avoid a duel. We have to balance being firm, yet gentle—almost casual. Your child is an individual and might not achieve mastery of this function at the same age as the child of your friend, who gains bragging rights about her toddler's accomplishment. Start with the right equipment—a potty-chair. Avoid the toddler seat that is affixed atop the standard toilet. I am certain that some toddlers, who have observed what happens to what is deposited in a standard toilet, would feel that they could be danger of going down the drain themselves while sitting atop one of these high monstrosities. Another drawback to this design is that a toddler will never be able to voluntarily get in "performance position" without help. I have witnessed stark fear in toddlers who are forcibly placed on one of these double-deckers, much the same as a four year old put in a barber's chair of dizzying height.

When the toddler acknowledges that he has something in his pants or diaper; this is a beginning. Pick your own word for bowel movement and stick with it. The next step is when the child can let you know when the action is going down. Practice anytime, just trying the potty-chair on for size to gain the comfort that develops the thought that this is *my* chair, for only me to use. When you, the parent, think you have picked up the "ready" signal, walk, don't run to the potty, take down the diaper or training pants, and see what happens. If nothing happens, dress the child up again. Give the process a little time, but avoid making it imperative that there is no way to get off the potty other than through a successful performance. When he or she does get up and is running around again, a bowel movement might soon follow. Chalk it up to a learning experience. If this happens frequently, it might indicate that inadvertently, expectations are too high. When the pressure is off, the anal sphincter relaxes.

The psychiatrist Sigmund Freud had much to say about "anal retention." We later labeled those suffering from this disorder as being "uptight." One doesn't hear much about Freudian theory any more. Medication has pretty much replaced the couch. But if you watch old movies, you will notice how many amateur psychiatrists there were in movies of the mid-1930s and 1940s, and how the plot of the movie was based on some Freudian theory. Fortunately Freud didn't seem to go further with application of his theories to infants or toddlers other than this concept of anal retention. As a pre-med student, I took every psych course I could squeeze in—general psychology, abnormal psychology, and child psychology. The abnormal psychology text read like a novel. Fascinating stuff. It caused students to see a bit of weirdness in themselves and, particularly, in their fellow classmates. Child psychology wasn't so "far out." It was more of what we have discussed—firm guidance, administered with love, and practiced consistently.

If a trainee ever regards a bowel movement as a worthy possession that he (almost exclusively "he") wants to keep or to prevent from being lost forever in some underground reservoir, we have a rougher road ahead. We have to avoid any resemblance of punishment for lack of proficiency and remember that bowel training is a learned process. Little successes are rewarded with loving praise. To avoid making bowel training a bigger issue than it deserves to be, it is probably best to not do much more than offer verbal praise. (Dispensing candy as a reward is definitely a poor idea.) Accidents happen. Voluntarily heading for the potty, whether or not in time, should be rewarded, as it is certainly a step in the right direction. When he begins to get the picture that a bowel movement is imminent, training pants are a big aid to independence. He can get through the preliminaries all by himself. If no breakthrough is forthcoming, examination is necessary to rule in or out several anatomical problems that could cause a toddler to seem to be holding back. To sum it up, avoid making a big deal of toilet training, thereby avoiding frustration that can further a defiant attitude.

The other side of the coin is exemplified by the following anecdote. I read of this in a pediatric journal in the 1960s, which was a time when many parents were terribly concerned about later-life consequences from bowel training. In a remote African village, the native children wore next to nothing and the infants nothing. Communal living was in buildings like long houses with dirt floors. By necessity, in the interest of maintaining minimal sanitation standards, slightly older children "trained" their infant siblings by the age of six months. There was some reference to the method, but it was pretty vague. Young children seemed to pick up signals from an infant in whom a bowel movement was just around the corner, apparently in the much same manner that some dogs learn the ability to detect that their master is on the verge of an epileptic seizure. The older sibling knew when to go with the infant to a "safe" place and somehow convey, possibly by stroking the infant's tummy, that now was the time. The message from this is that bowel control *had* to happen, and it did, without the application of any pressure or any sense of failure.

Abnormalities of the stool itself can usually be taken care of easily. Constipation can come from too little fiber in the diet or the food itself, often due to milk allergy. (See the allergy chapter.) A good intake of beneficial bacteria is helpful. B vitamins aid the tone of the intestinal tract. Half of a B50, in two doses spread throughout the day, ground up and put in juice or in a bite of food, followed by more of the food without the "additive," should help. Anything further should be prescribed only after examination and might include a detergentlike stool softener. If a constipated stool sits in the rectum for too long a period, relief might have to come from a small Ducolax enema until the cause is determined. This problem needs correction, because attempting to pass a hard, good-sized stool can create an anal fissure (tear) that can become painful and make the next attempt to pass a hard stool much more difficult—something to be avoided.

Sleep Problems

It has long been my principle to look for simple causes first. A medical school professor admonished our far-reaching student responses to his questions on medical (educational) rounds. He said to us, "Your trouble is, when you hear hoof beats, you think of zebras." Before pursuing the diagnosis of the uncommon, think of the common first.

Children grow fast and the need for nourishment, hardwired into each of us, is especially dramatic in babies. Hunger can be a mighty powerful reason for a baby waking frequently during the night. Often, the infant is just plain hungry, or there is milk or food intolerance. My coauthor, Dr. Saul, told me of his own observation. His infant son was getting hospital-recommended infant formula to "supplement" breast-feeding. The infant formula apparently caused a tummy ache—with symptoms indistinguishable from those of hunger—and the parents wisely returned to exclusive breast-feeding. Problem solved.

Unlike an adult with sleep problems, an infant's problem is not "in his head," with few exceptions. Some active infants insist on a "terra firma" sleep position with their backs firmly against a crib side bumper or on their tummy, with legs drawn up, on a firm mattress. Some, seemingly too immature to be able to, can be seen to scoot up to end of the crib in order to get their heads firmly against the boundary marking headboard.

The SIDS prevention doctrine gives little room for considering these positions, but I see no reason not to satisfy this desire as long as the bumpers are solid and firmly fixed, and if the mattress and bedding are rendered unable to obstruct the infant's airway. Many pediatricians feel that the "back to sleep" program is inviolable. Discuss this with your doctor if you have an insistent infant. I think the choice should be yours—it's your final decision.

If sleep comes with difficulty to an infant, we adults have to scratch our heads and try to figure out why. An infant is not going to purposely stay awake in order to keep us awake. Something is wrong. Before going to the doctor, be armed with knowledge gained from some detective work. Is there discomfort from an upset bowel, as revealed by a distended abdomen, passing gas, or a messy bowel movement? Or is the problem higher up, stomach discomfort revealed by frequent spitting-up accompanied by crying. Or is it with both bowel and stomach, showing an association with feeding or specific ingredients of the feeding.

Pain from an earache may not seem to be related to the ear in an infant. It should be a suspect if the baby has signs of a cold, or cold and fever, or just wants to be held in an upright position (to reduce throbbing pain) and holds one side of the head close to a body. Discomfort from an earache makes sleep nearly impossible. Restlessness results from pain. We can presume that infants might suffer from the same aches and pains that adults have during a viral infectious illness. The presence of fever increases the chance that the restlessness is associated with minor aches and pains. Since an infant is unable to describe what is going on, a doctor visit is in order to rule out a more serious problem if there are signs of sickness such as undue restlessness and irritability or listlessness and being "off of feeding." For infants, fever can be of no consequence or a marker of a bacterial infection that requires immediate evaluation and treatment.

Unlike an infant whose sleep problems are related more to physical (somatic) factors, the toddler is more affected by what is going on in his or her developing brain (psychic factors). Many of the solutions for sleep problems parallel those for adults: (1) Prepare for sleep. Start ahead of the designated sleep time by reducing sensory stimuli, such as turning off the television, having the whole family engage in only quiet activity, dimming or turning off lights. Spend some limited time at crib side with comforting words, or with the older toddler, try a quieting bedside story. (2) If a gap has somehow opened between when *you* want your child to call it a day and what time your toddler thinks it should be, close the gap by increments. Daylight savings time (here to stay), in either "springing forward" or "falling back," creates a sixty-minute discrepancy—too large to correct in one night. So go about the correction in increments—ten or fifteen minutes per night. Darkening the room might be needed. (3) If the child is waking up during the night, first do as you would do with an infant—look for a physical cause. If there is no noticeable physical cause and the child awakens with crying, consider the possibility of a bad dream. A toddler can usually express what scared him. If he shows stark fear with trembling and a vacant stare and has no idea of why he is in this state, he might have had a night terror episode, which is more serious than a nightmare. Night terrors are very disturbing to the toddler and observer alike. The reason this less common condition occurred must be investigated, because some severe psychologically stressful event is at the root of this reaction. (4) Sometimes a cry can be answered with just a reassuring word that all is well. More often, a parent will have to go to the bedside to administer comfort. Make sure to give only enough comfort as promptly as possible to fill the bill, to avoid setting a pattern.

Spanking

Much is said and written about corporal punishment. For infants, with no concept of wrongdoing, it is a *non sequitur*. Spanking or any other kind of so-called "corporal punishment" of an infant has to be considered totally and utterly inappropriate. Strangely enough, when cases of child (infant) abuse are evaluated, the abuser usually simply, but mistakenly, thinks he or she is administering discipline. This creates a conundrum for social workers. A social worker's job is to investigate and attempt to eliminate child abuse. First of all, they must have a fair evaluation of the motives of the abuser. Did a well-intentioned person simply get carried away with an immature concept of discipline? If so, that person needs to be counseled to stop and can reasonably be expected to so do. But if it is a case of clear and present danger, crisis management is in order.

The spanking issue gets stickier when we consider what to do with a naughty, or defiant, or impulsive, or strong-willed, or all-of-the-above, toddler. It's almost like debating capital punishment; each position has its pros and its cons. "Spare the rod and spoil the child" versus "Hopefully, the little demon will grow out of this bad behavior." Perhaps the biblical "rod" is not an instrument that inflicts pain, but is more like the shepherd's staff that comforts by providing the security of limits on behavior. Sorry, complete permissiveness will not make problems simply disappear. It will reinforce them. We have to get beyond the concept of "punishment" and think of "discipline" (teaching) instead. Fit the disciplinary action to the toddler's ability to understand what it is all about. If quick action is needed to side step danger, and the person who disciplines can put aside any anger, I *suppose* a quick swat on the buttocks might be in order. I have to admit I am not squarely in the "spare the rod" camp, but I would hope to concoct a workable peace plan before calling for war. If a parent ever *has* to resort to spanking, there must be a sincere effort afterwards to convey the fact that the punishment was administered with love. This requires a lot of skill. A very advanced child will think, "Oh sure. What kind of hypocrisy is this? You say it hurts *you* more than it hurts *me*."

The authors, and most of the authors' contemporaries, were raised when spanking was routine and quite beyond discussion. In this way, the good old days weren't. Decades ago, when I (AWS) was a young parent, I spanked my children. I regret it to this day. Fortunately, becoming a teacher wised me up. Even in the 1980s, corporal punishment had already long been extinguished in most school systems. That is good. Teachers simply must, by law, learn and administer nonphysical, nonviolent discipline. My experience as an educator showed me what I was slow to learn as a parent: Creative behavior management works, and works well.

But you have to have the moxie to actually do it. Things as they are may be getting out of hand. Today, many, *many* schools are in desperate need of discipline. Teacher inaction and administrative leniency are being substituted for nonphysical but consistently enforced discipline. I once worked in a tough urban public school where the administration ignored everything except huge discipline problems. The result? They only *had* huge problems, and lots of them. The disciplinary administrator's waiting room looked like an overcrowded pet shop fish tank. Kids were literally standing sardines, packed in and pressed against the glass window.

Another time, I worked in a parochial system. Relax: The only nuns with rulers were art teachers or technology teachers, and no knuckles were touched at any time, ever. I asked a parochial school administrator what her biggest discipline problem was. She thought for a long moment, and then answered: "Gum chewing." Don't chuckle for too long. If you care about the small stuff, the big stuff doesn't happen. And don't try to tell me that "all the kids in parochial schools are angels." I taught at quite a variety of schools. Parochial school

REWARDING GOOD BEHAVIOR

Over the years, I (AWS) have worked for a number of school administrators. One of the best principals I know had a sign in his office that read, "Really surprise someone today: Catch them doing something right." I saw this and knew I was in the right place. It is a great philosophy for educators, and it is very practical tactic for parents. When toddlers (or children of any age, really) are playing quietly by themselves and "being good," that is not the time for you to make a phone call, get work done, or even to sit and relax. Yes, those things may well need doing. But this is your moment to accomplish something greater: this is *the* time to go to your child, unbidden, and praise them openly. Sit down with them. Tell them just how impressed you are. Offering positive attention for peaceful, self-directed constructive activity rewards it. Reward the behavior you want, and you will get more of it. Speak up and praise the quiet behavior and you will get even more responsible behavior than that. There is pretty much nothing a small child wants more than adult approval and personal attention. Catch them doing something good, and you head off having to respond to something bad.

So many years ago, before I became a "regular" teacher, I substitute-taught a second grade class. At the front of the room was an isolated desk, occupied sporadically by a hyperactive, blatantly defiant, loud child. All the children knew why he was there, and it took only seconds for me to get my on-the-spot briefing. He would climb out of his seat, stand up, wander, talk out of turn, interrupt, disturb other children, and generally acted out obnoxiously. So I started to personally address the children around him. I said, "I really like the way you are sitting!" to one settled, attentive child. To another very quiet child, I said, "You are looking like you are ready to work. That's great!" Out of the corner of my eye, I saw the Kid from Hades watching it all, standing and leaning like a racehorse ready to bolt but tentatively thinking it over first. Then I asked the class questions. The kids that blurted out answers I ignored, and I only called on children with their hands raised. In only a short time, I noticed out of the corner of my eye that the Boy in the "Special" Seat was sitting square in his chair, at his desk, and looking at me. Then I asked the class another question. I saw his hand rocket up in reply, and I instantly rounded on him, saying, "Yes? What would *you* like to say?" I had no further difficulty from him, and he was engaged the whole class.

Good child management displaces the craving, yea the drive, for any attention at any price. Catch them doing something right. The effort it takes is a blue-chip investment in a happier day for the child, and for you.

students had the same pack of problems that their public-schooled neighbors had.

Some public school teachers do, or try to do, a superb job with discipline. Really good teachers I knew used delightfully clever and effective methods. One teacher had errant students surrender one of the shoes or sneakers until class was over. It worked. The teacher was ordered by the front office to stop. In another district, there was a teacher who had "Detention with Old Blue Eyes." Kids who stayed after school for him had to listen to his Frank Sinatra records. There were complaints; he too was ordered to stop.

Dr. Campbell was on his local school board with a marvelous superintendent, who put a stop to the little transgressions that prevented greater ones. His methods trickled down to principals who backed their teachers. The schools and students thrived. But that superintendent was followed by a passive guy that seemed to figure that kids didn't need discipline or even guidance—that they would magically come out all right. The downhill course was unimaginable. Conscientious teachers had no backing, and students picked up on this fast. And without help at home, where discipline should be started very early in the child's life, a teacher just can't do it all.

Hitting is wrong no matter who does it, and two wrongs will never, ever make a right. I say this having no moral ascendency. I am in no position to look down on anyone. Truth is, I learned *later* that spanking is reprehensible. I *first* learned that not spanking my kids got better results, by far, than spanking them. I would use the old 1-2-3 counting system, take away their television time, ground them for part of the day, or levy fines against their allowance. Anything but corporal punishment. One of my children once actually appealed my nonviolent sentence, and requested a spanking in order to have the day free. I declined. Teaching had taught the teacher to be a better parent.

SUMMARY

Good patterns for successful living as an adult are instilled early in life. Parents, pick your objectives early, begin early, and be consistent. As the adult and being wiser, do what you think is right, always accompanied with a show of love. Be on the alert for signs of understanding and the chance to help your child substitute reasoning for blind obedience. The strong-willed child poses more of a challenge. But keeping that active brain and body under control without dampening spirits, can be rewarding later on. Hang in there and enjoy.

CHAPTER 13

SUDDEN INFANT DEATH
SYNDROME (SIDS)

SIDS is defined as unexpected sudden death in an infant, or crib death. "Unexpected," in that there had been no prior detected health problems in the infant. Could anything be more devastating to parents than this? Their precious one, seemingly in good health when put down for sleep, only to later be found lifeless. Infants are felt to be vulnerable between three and twelve months of age—the end of infancy.

When this first became a medical diagnosis appearing in the medical literature in the 1960s, it was an unknown to most, even in the medical profession. To compound the tragedy, many parents were accused, sometimes outrightly, of abusing their infant. If the accusation was not derived from direct physical evidence, then there was the implication of parental neglect of some sort as searching for the cause began. Even today, there are many suspects of contributors, even if only tangential, to causes of the syndrome—keeping the baby too warm, exposure to tobacco smoke, being related to premature birth, (with all sorts of reasons given as the cause of the prematurity)—even relating it to obscure descriptions of "neural architecture" that controls breathing, or "abnormal signal transaction."

My observation, which fortunately is limited, is that inexplicable grief immediately raises the question of "why," followed (without getting an answer to the first question) by, "What did I do wrong?" The feeling of guilt is palpable. Even a very skillful, empathetic doctor or other examiner attempting to make sense out of this seemingly

185

senseless situation will unwittingly increase the guilt feelings, as questions pertaining to possible causes are entertained.

Originally, the diagnosis of SIDS was one of exclusion of previously undiscovered health problems. This can only be done by a careful autopsy, performed by a qualified pediatric pathologist (as is even still required today). A definitive diagnosis resulted from the finding of "petichiae in the mediastinum." In nonmedical terms, little blood spots in the tissue surrounding the trachea (the mediastinum) appear after a strong, last-ditch effort at breathing in, when laryngospasm has thoroughly sealed off the top of the windpipe. When the windpipe is blocked off, a tremendous effort to pull air into the lungs (an agonal gasp) follows. This strong expansion of the chest cavity while the airway is blocked creates negative pressure in the chest and literally pulls red blood cells out of the small capillary blood vessels of the mediastinum to the surface. All of this describes the known cause of death, but it doesn't explain what caused the laryngospasm in the first place.

It would be reasonable to think that a parent would want to know exactly what caused this terrible tragedy. But giving permission for some medical super-specialist, found only in a large metropolitan area, to operate on a loved one's lifeless body, is nearly impossible for many as they suffer such overwhelming grief. Consequently, various causes of suffocation muddied the waters. A "pure" diagnosis was not sought many times. At present, the specificity of diagnosis is being diluted by making SIDS a subset of a broader SUID category (a Centers for Disease Control and Prevention [CDC] term)—SUID standing for "sudden unexplained infant deaths." I don't think a name change in itself changes much because, after a thorough investigation of an infant death, obvious causes of asphyxiation are often uncovered which provide a clear cause of death. This still leaves the cause of the agonal laryngospasm of true SIDS unsolved.

In 1992, after pursuing all possible theories of the cause of SIDS, the American Academy of Pediatrics (AAP) felt they had a significant finding: Data gathering indicated that infants who sleep on their tummies (prone position) are much more apt to succumb to SIDS. From the beginning of AAP's SIDS prevention efforts whether or not intentionally, they were describing the broader category, SUID, as prone-positioned babies were more apt to obstruct their airways from soft bedding or to wiggle over to crib sides that could entrap their heads. One theory was that for some reason these babies had a problem similar to "sleep apnea," in which they would simply stop breathing. Right there they got away from the original concept of the basic pathology of SIDS. By doing so they heaped unimaginable anxiety on parents. Normal infants with a sibling who had succumbed to SIDS were hooked up to an apnea monitor. If the infant momentarily stopped breathing during sleep, an alarm designed to alert the parent would go off. The frantic, untrained parent was somehow expected to get the infant breathing again. Eventually, this idea was abandoned and replaced by the Back to Sleep campaign (now called the Safe to Sleep campaign) that put the emphasis on sleep position.

Several of us pediatricians who were "in the trenches" questioned the SIDS committee concerning their recommendation to *always* put an infant down for sleep on its back. We illustrated our position by describing a newborn with choanal atresia. This is a rare condition in which a newborn's nasal passages have not fully developed and are not open all the way into the back of the throat. Until these babies have an operation to open the airway, they can only be kept alive by someone stimulating them to mouth-breathe. As soon as they fall asleep, they simply won't breathe without this stimulation (such as tickling the nose with a wisp of cotton). The baby with this condition is the extreme example of being an obligatory nose breather—a condition shared by all infants that disappears, with some individual variation, as the infant's nervous system matures. Also, with a relatively common respiratory infection due to an adenovirus that causes a very stuffy (blocked) nose, an infant can produce an unfathomable amount of "gunk" (there is no better word) in the back of the throat, where the nasal airway enters. In an adult, we call this postnasal drip. A baby flat on its back simply can not get out of the way of this deluge and chokes and gags until it can. The same thing is true concerning getting out of the way of vomitus. Even if not vomiting, just spitting up while in the on-the-back position can be problematic.

Another side issue is the development of a misshapen head (medical term: plagiocephaly). With normal growth, the skull volume increases to accommodate a growing brain, but that volume can occupy many different shapes of cranial vaults. A baby constantly kept on its back develops a noticeably flattened head, which can be accompanied with frontal bossing, or bulging of the forehead.

SIDS supporters argued that babies couldn't get out of the prone position when they needed to and thus be apt to jam the nose and mouth into the bedding. I don't agree. When supported by the examiner's hand under the belly a normal active newborn, only a few hours old, will automatically put her hands down and turn her head to the side as she makes "a soft landing" facing down. An active baby only a few months of age, who might later be said to suffer from ADHD, will often scoot up the crib until his head is firmly against the headboard (or pad) when he is put down prone.

Our efforts to point out drawbacks to the program were in vain. Full speed ahead! Pediatricians were continuously alerted. AAP headquarters even sent little signs that were to be placed in infant examining rooms, urging parents to ask the doctor about sleeping position. Probably the main benefit of the program was that the infants were being examined by a knowledgeable doctor or assistant, who imparted other related tips on how to avoid SIDS or SUIDS, more as a spin-off of the main thrust of promoting sleeping on the back. Suspected contributing factors might be discussed and parents would be told to avoid soft bedding, including soft crib-side pads; avoid exposure to tobacco smoke; avoid overdressing or too much bundling that allows body temperature to rise; check with your doctor if there is any hint of an illness; and so on.

To the AAP's credit, they recognized the need to impart this education, a need that was not being met. A drawback to Social Service Medicare programs was that mothers were not encouraged to seek out medical care superior to that obtained from an emergency center—making a mockery of the word "emergency." An emergency center is only going to provide acute care, and even that is often deficient in quality. For instance, when diagnosing and treating an earache, the emergency room (ER) doctor is handicapped by not knowing the patient's medical history. And probably a habitual ER patron knows very little of it either. So the need to provide care to infants from someone who could be called the infant's doctor, someone who could keep a medical record and provide helpful health education, was apparent.

Consequently, there was a sweeping movement in California to do just that. Many new Well Clinics were started. Referrals from social service agencies and other programs such as the Women's, Infants', Children's (WIC) program dramatically increased the numbers of clinic clients. Incentives to participate in this new type of healthcare included having food vouchers from WIC tied to attending a well clinic. These two government-subsidized programs provided a lot more bang for the financial buck than random ER visits. Clients, of course, had no concern about the cost of either program. Basically, all kinds of health problems could be revealed by a comprehensive examination. In this setting, clients would be much more apt to listen, not only to the back-to-sleep message, but also to all the spin-off suggestions we mentioned. Other health education was provided, varying from clinic to clinic—on rare occasions, even nutrition education. Clinics rapidly popped up everywhere.

SIDS AND VITAMIN C DEFICIENCY

> "If the Vitamin C status of an infant is borderline, the administration of a vaccine, particularly (but not only) pertussis vaccine, can result in endotoxaemia. This results in a severe reaction to the vaccine, a tremendous increase in the need for Vitamin C, and the precipitation of some of the signs and/or symptoms of acute scurvy. The onset of this may be so rapid that the classical signs of scurvy may be absent. Sudden death, sudden unconsciousness, sudden shock or sudden spontaneous bruising and haemorrhage (including brain and retinal haemorrhages) may occur. Haemorrhage and bruising in such cases can be wrongly attributed to the 'battered baby syndrome.'"[1]
>
> —ARCHIE KALOKERINOS, M.D.

I kibitzed on the Mr. H. case—a case in which the father was accused of (and looking at an ominous sentence for) the "shaken baby syndrome," which allegedly leads to tearing cerebral vessels from their moorings and leads to brain death. The best evidence of it is the detection of retinal hemorrhages. Dr. Kalokerinos was called as an expert witness and made an excellent case for hemorrhaging due to scurvy (shaking or not). The endotoxin theory was not mentioned, nor was it needed; the mother had suffered from pernicious nausea of pregnancy for most of her pregnancy and was very poorly nourished, herself. The defense jumped on the pediatrician (and I thought, justly so) for having giving this obviously puny, premature baby a "routine" diphtheria, whooping cough, and tetanus (DPT) shot at the first visit. Dr. Kalokerinos convinced me and many others that the stress of this vaccination further depleted the baby's minimal vitamin C reserves to the point of bleeding in the brain and retinae occurred, without the need of violent shaking. His vast amount of experience, in which he gave vitamin C whenever he administered a vaccination, backed his testimony. Other factors, like an autopsy report that was for another infant, got Mr. H. acquitted from the serious accusation, but everyone learned a great deal about vitamin C deficiency in relationship to receiving a vaccination, particularly a DPT.

ARCHIE KALOKERINOS, M.D. (1927–2012)
Orthomolecular Medicine Hall of Fame 2009

"Any attempt to adequately write about Archie Kalokerinos would need a thousand pages and would incorporate many such adjectives as: far-sighted, intelligent, sensible, observant, honest, caring, altruistic, congenial, meticulous, brave, dogged, intrepid, and last but not least, the trite, but well-deserved, 'great.'"

—OSCAR FALCONI

Archivides "Archie" Kalokerinos was born in Glenn Innes, Australia, in 1927 and took his M.D. degree from Sydney University in 1951.

He was appointed Medical Superintendent of the hospital at Collarenebri, Australia, where he served until 1975. His practice is based on Linus Pauling's theory that many diseases result from excessive free radicals and can accordingly be prevented or cured by vitamin C.

Kalokerinos is well known worldwide as the doctor who spent much of his time fighting for the well-being of the Aboriginal inhabitants of Australia. He became very concerned about the high death rate of Aboriginal children in New South Wales and came to the conclusion that the infants had symptoms of scurvy, a deficiency of vitamin C. In his ground-breaking book, *Every Second Child,*[1] he discovered that the an acute vitamin C deficiency provoked by the vaccinations was the reason why, at a certain point, up to half of the vaccinated Aboriginal infants died. Instead of being rewarded for this lifesaving observation, Kalokerinos was harassed and his methods were disregarded by the authorities, probably because they were too simple, too cheap, and too efficacious to be accepted by the vested interests of modern medicine. And, besides, they were meant to protect a population which, in its own native county, is regarded by some as not worth taking the trouble for anyway. Dr. Kalokerinos, however, thought differently, and the Nobel Prize winner Linus Pauling (who wrote the foreword to *Every Second Child*) endorsed his views.

Kalokerinos was a Life Fellow of the Royal Society for the Promotion of Health, the International Academy of Preventive Medicine, the Australian College of Biomedical Scientists, the Hong Kong Medical Technology Association, and a Member of the New York Academy of Sciences. In 1978 he was awarded the Australian Medal of Merit (AMM) for outstanding scientific research. He is an author of twenty-eight papers listed in PubMed. He retired from full-time practice in 1993 and devoted the rest of his life to private research.

Reference

1. Kalokerinos, A. *Every Second Child*. Melbourne, Australia: Thomas Nelson (Australia) Ltd., 1974.

Dr. Kalokerinos makes rather sweeping statements, and he might very well be right. He said, "When I discovered that immunizations were dangerous, [I] achieved a substantial drop in death rate." But then he had already discovered and exercised what he had learned concerning how vitamin C, given just prior to an immunization procedure, reduced the toxicity. Dr. Kalokerinos had a vast experience with vitamin C and the DPT vaccination, and he may very well be right in applying that knowledge to *all* immunizations.

He said, "If endotoxin is the cause of otitis and also cause of SIDS, sudden unexplained unconsciousness and unexplained shock—as I now know (at least there is an association)—then otitis media should be found in a significant number of SIDS cases. This is clearly demonstrated in a number of studies."

My (RKC) experience tells me that endotoxin as a cause of otitis media (OM) or SIDS and related neurological abnormalities is not clearly demonstrated. I have not seen such studies, although I would not rule out the possibility of them having been kept out side the mainstream—much like Abram Hoffer's and other orthomolecutlar medicine doctors' works. There are always pathogens lurking in the nasopharynx. With the partial vacuum formed with Eustachian tube blockage, bacteria are literally sucked into the middle ear space where they multiply nicely in the hypoxic, warm environment. The main cause of OM is blockage. Certainly endotoxins in the system could not be the cause of SIDS. If sticking to the pathognomonic laryngospasm finding, I find it hard to see how a blood-borne endotoxin would selectively exert its effect on the larynx. I don't think Dr. Kalokerinos sees it that way either when he mentions "shock"—we know how gram-negative organisms (but these gram-negative shock-producing organisms are not common pathogens related to OM) can produce toxins that cause septic shock—and other nervous system problems. Unless both OM and SIDS are caused by endotoxin, we won't find studies relating the two. He tones this down with "at least there is an association." In an infant, the first sign of OM is fussiness. By definition, SIDS victims are deemed well by their parents when they are put down to sleep.

Let us be careful to continue to think about what this brilliant man had to say, but let's not give the impression that he has the final answer in the search for a cause of SIDS. Research continues in this area. Let it be pointed and honest—not diluted by accepting tangential causes that can not explain the root cause, laryngeal spasm. Dr. Kalokerinos's experience showing the value of giving vitamin C before an immunization is given, has proven very beneficial. Vitamin C deficiency has been suspected as a cause of SIDS for over seventy years, and clearly implicated as the cause for over twenty years. A number of scientific articles are available on this topic, many of which are available on the Internet.[2]

THE DECREASE IN SIDS

The first evaluation of the Back to Sleep campaign that was published in *Pediatrics,* the journal of the AAP, was a California study. Data was gathered from the new clinics. The authors of the study concluded that what was causing a dramatic drop in SIDS incidence was based entirely on sleeping position—avoiding the prone and encouraging the supine position. Side issues, such as the benefits mentioned above, were not considered significant, although they were to continue being a part of health education given in the well clinics. Pediatricians were continuously notified of dangers that predispose to SUID that superseded those already in vogue (not necessarily pure SIDS), such as faulty cribs in which the side could inadvertently fall down on the child's head or body, too-soft crib bumpers, and sleeping in bed with mother. Surely, explaining these dangers to the clinic clients would have had some impact on lowering the incidence of SIDS or SUID.

The latest advice is to put the infant asleep with a pacifier. If it is spit out, don't reinsert it. *The mechanism is unknown,* but nevertheless this is the recommendation. Many studies describe a reduced incidence of SIDS in nursing babies. Other studies state that there is an increased risk of SIDS with babies in bed with their nursing mother. It would seem that nursing and sleeping should be separated. Don't simulate nursing by sticking a pacifier in the baby's mouth. The nursing model (nature's way) does not suggest that a baby should be constantly sucking. At the same time, the upright position provided from an infant seat (or portable car seat) is now condemned.

CONCLUSION

Early on, it was considered safe for a baby to be placed on its side as a sleep position. This was abandoned, and stricter enforcement of placing the infant on its back ensued. Supervised (an adult nearby) "tummy time" was suggested. *Watch that infant every second or the little dickens might get in serious trouble.* My goodness! How did previous generations ever survive? All this attention by the AAP to sleep position detracts from the search for deeper causes and puts a parent in the awkward and puzzling position of deciding whom to listen to—the voice of authority, or the voice of common sense? I suggest listening to and carefully considering all the warnings your doctor provides and then evaluate your infant's motor abilities as he seeks a comfortable position on a firm surface (no loose bedding). Does he easily avoid obstructing his mouth and nose and move to keep his airway free when on his tummy? Unfortunately, the practicing pediatrician has to stick with the Safe to Sleep campaign, putting any idea of choice squarely on backs of the parents. Interestingly, the earlier name "Back to Sleep" was recently changed to "Safe to Sleep." So much of the emphasis had been put on the importance of sleep position—making it the *prime* causal factor—that the significance of all the other factors that came under the umbrella of "undecided" (SUIDS) got little attention. Perhaps the name change resulted from experts "seeing the light," leading to improved health education. Let's hope so.

CHAPTER 14

HIGH-DOSE VITAMIN C THERAPY FOR YOUNG CHILDREN

Although we hope you will read through this whole chapter, here is the executive summary: Vitamin C is the single most important, and most often overlooked, therapeutic nutrient for babies and small children. Children need more vitamin C than the government says they do. Sick children need even more, far more. Bowel tolerance is the guideline for therapeutic use of vitamin C. Bowel tolerance means exactly what you think it means. Loose stool indicates vitamin C saturation. We are not advocating diarrhea. Loose, soft stool is *not* watery, explosive diarrhea. If a child already has loose stool, vitamin C will usually, paradoxically, improve it. Because vitamin C is antiviral, it is likely to help stop diarrhea. The way to check is to simply back off the dose: if the looseness goes away, then it was too much C. Now keep the child at saturation by adjusting the dose as needed. Symptoms come back: give more C. Stool too loose: give less C. Symptoms stay away and stool is good: just right. Take enough C to be symptom free, whatever the amount might be. This is a self-adjusting technique. As the child gets better, he or she will automatically hold less vitamin C.

PUTTING THE "C" IN CURE

What is it about a little left-handed molecule made up of six carbon, six oxygen, and eight hydrogen atoms that ticks off so many in the medical community? Maybe it's cases like this one: Ray, a health professional I (AWS) know, had an eleven-month-old son who was very sick for over a week. No one, and I mean no one, in their family had had any sleep in a long time. They were up night after night with this child, who had a high fever, glazed watery eyes, tons of thick watery mucus, and labored breathing. The child would not sleep, and did little else but cry. The baby was under the care of a pediatrician, who, in the infant's eleven months on earth, had already prescribed twelve rounds of some very serious antibiotics. It was all too apparent to Ray that they were not working. Out of desperation he decided to try something he previously had been taught *not* to try: bowel-tolerance quantities of oral ascorbate. Ray and his wife gave their baby vitamin C about every fifteen minutes. As a result, the baby noticeably improved in a matter of hours, and slept through the night. With continuing frequent doses the child was completely well in less than forty-eight hours. Ray calculated that the child had received just over 2,000 mg vitamin C per kilogram body weight per day. This is even more than what vitamin C expert Dr. Frederick Robert Klenner customarily ordered for sick patients. Remarkably, at 20,000 milligrams of vitamin C per day, Ray's baby never had bowel-tolerance loose stools.[1]

You have to marvel at where all that ascorbate was going in such a little body. Of course, it is the opinion of those who promulgate the U.S. Recommended Dietary Allowance (RDA) and related nutritional mythology that almost all of that baby's vitamin C went uselessly into the toilet. Ray and his wife would tell you differently. They would say that their sick child soaked it up like a sponge, and then promptly got better. You choose the answer that works for you.

QUANTITY AND FREQUENCY OF DOSE ARE THE KEYS TO ASCORBATE THERAPY

Dr. Frederick Robert Klenner earned his M.D. from Duke University School of Medicine and was subsequently board certified in diseases of the chest.[2] A working summation of Dr. Klenner's therapeutic use of vitamin C is 350 milligrams of vitamin C per kilogram of body weight per day (350 mg/kg/day), in divided doses.[3] Since a kilogram is about 2.2 pounds, this translates as shown in the following chart.

MILLIGRAMS OF VITAMIN C	BODY WEIGHT	NUMBER OF DOSES	AMOUNT PER DOSE
35,000 mg	220 lb	17–18	2,000 mg
18,000 mg	110 lb	18	1,000 mg
9,000 mg	55 lb	18	500 mg
4,500 mg	28 lb	9	500 mg
2,300 mg	14–15 lb	9	250 mg
1,200 mg	7–8 lb	9	130–135 mg

Although these quantities may seem high, *Dr. Klenner actually used as much as four times these amounts for serious viral illness,* administered by injection. The oral doses listed above are, for the doctor, comparatively moderate.

Vitamin supplements are much safer than medicines, so it is not necessary to be that exact in figuring how much to give. With our kids, we found it convenient to think, "What fraction of an adult do we have here?" We figured an adult dose for an adult weight. If an adult was 180 pounds and one tablet, then a 90-pound adolescent was half a tablet and a 45-pound child was one-quarter tablet. One-eighth tablet would be fine for a 23-pound toddler and one-sixteenth tablet for a baby of 12 pounds. You can safely round up and give more than this. Pound for pound, a youngster's need for vitamins is proportionally greater than that of an adult.

Frequency of Dose

Injections of vitamin C may be arranged with your physician. For those unable to obtain intravenous vitamin C, it is essential to pay special attention to one of the most important aspects of vitamin C therapy: *Dividing the dosage improves absorption and retention of vitamin C.* High oral doses of vitamin C yield higher blood levels of the vitamin, and dividing the oral doses maintains those higher levels. Although initially it may seem almost too obvious to mention, these are not self-evident concepts. Many medical website and government-based dietary recommendations hinge on ignoring them. Hilary Roberts, Ph.D., writes: "Stressed and even mildly ill people can tolerate 1,000 times more vitamin C, implying a change in biochemistry that was ignored in creating the RDA. In setting the RDA, unsubstantiated risks of taking too much vitamin C have been accorded great importance, whereas the risks of not taking enough have been ignored. Real scientists understand that 'no scientific proof' is a fancy way of saying 'we don't like this idea.'"[4]

And there is ample proof to not like. Vitamin C, in very high doses, has been used to successfully treat several dozen illnesses,[5] with published, peer-reviewed literature spanning the last sixty years. Therefore, the effectiveness and safety of megadose vitamin C therapy should, by now, be yesterday's news. Yet I never cease to be amazed at the number of persons who remain unaware that vitamin C is the best broad-spectrum antibiotic, antihistamine, antitoxic, and antiviral substance there is. Equally surprising is the ease with which some people, most of the medical profession, and virtually all of the media have been convinced that, somehow, vitamin C is not only ineffective but is also downright dangerous.

You may also give twice as many doses, with half as much C per dose. Vitamin C may be given as liquid, powder, tablet, or chewable tablet. Infants often prefer finely powdered, naturally sweetened chewable tablets, which can be crushed between two spoons. You can make your own liquid vitamin C by daily dissolving C powder in a small (one ounce) dropper bottle and adding a sweetener if necessary. Dr. Klenner of course recommended daily preventive doses, which might be about one-sixth of the above therapeutic amount. Preventive doses should be divided into three doses daily.

People with sensitivity to citrus fruits, tomatoes, or cranberries may feel more comfortable taking vitamin C as ascorbate, a non-acidic form of vitamin C. Calcium ascorbate is most frequently chosen and sodium ascorbate the least, except for injection. The transition down to a maintenance level (about 60 mg/kg/day) should be made gradually, over a period of a week or two.

Everyday Preventive Dosage Amounts

Pediatrician Lendon H. Smith, M.D., said, "Vitamin C is our best defense and everyone should be on this one even before birth. Three thousand milligrams daily for the pregnant woman is a start. The baby should get *100 mg per day per month of age.* (The six-month-old would get 600 mg, the year-old gets a thousand mgs daily, the two-year-old would get 2,000 mg, etc.) A daily dose of 2,000 to 5,000 mg would be prudent for a lifetime."

Dr. Klenner recommended daily preventive doses of 10,000 to 15,000 mg vitamin C per day. He advised parents to give their children their age in vitamin C grams (1 g = 1,000 mg). That would be 2,000 mg per day for a two-year-old, 9,000 mg per day for a nine-year-old, and for older children, a leveling off at about 10,000 mg per day. As for me, I simply say, "Take enough vitamin C to be symptom free, whatever that amount may be." It worked for my family.

After reading the account above of the sick baby that needed 20,000 milligrams of vitamin C to get well, many a reader has asked, "Exactly how do you get that much vitamin C into a baby?" Food supplements don't do much good in the bottle.

"So Where Can I Buy Liquid Vitamin C That Has a Really Good-Sized Dose to It?"

Beats me. Plus, I think you are better off making your own, fresh, every day. Liquid vitamin C is vitamin C dissolved in water, which is not very stable; potency is lost by the hour. On the other hand, vitamin C (ascorbic acid) powder is cheap and very stable (we're talking years here). You can buy it on the Internet.

So no, there's no need to wander the shopping malls hunting in vain for high-potency liquid vitamin C. Just take plain ascorbic acid crystals (available from any health food store, and many online suppliers), dissolve as much as you can in a given amount of water, and make your own.

HINTS TO GET INFANTS TO TAKE THEIR VITAMINS WITH A MINIMUM OF FUSS

Here are ways to make vitamin taking easier for your youngster.

Chewable and Liquid Vitamins

For little children, there are very tasty chewable vitamins and liquid preparations for infants. They usually taste yummy (try one!) and are readily accepted by most kids. Liquid vitamin preparations have two drawbacks. One is that the potencies tend to be low. Well, babies tend to be little, so no big deal. Two, they do not keep particularly well after opening, and they lose potency quickly even in the refrigerator. However, they are easiest to administer to infants.

Alternatively, and especially for toddlers, you can try pulverizing a chewable into a fine powder. Crush it between two spoons, and then put in half-spoonful of a sweet food. This does not guarantee instant success, though. With young-uns, no matter what you give or how you give it, it may still come burbling out and end up on the floor, on the highchair or on you. Try it again. It's just like learning to walk. As it becomes routine, the child will accept it. Start early and acceptance will come early. Good habits thus formed will bring dividends for years.

A Spoonful of Sugar?

Of course, children's chewable vitamin C may be delicious, but they are pricey. As an alumnus of the "Mary Poppins School of Medicine," let me say that the answer is sugar. Pure ascorbic acid dissolved in sugar water is the cheapest "solution" there is. Yes, sugar, that universal bane of health writers. Sweet, sweet sugar is the way to get little kids to take tons of sour, sour ascorbic acid.

Now I am *not* suggesting that you gorge your offspring on sugar. I'm simply a realist. Sugar is cheap, and it works. And it works with sick kids at 3:00 A.M. Putting vitamin C powder in really sweet natural fruit juice often does the trick, too.

Dosing Hints

Hint 1: *Rinse after.* Because vitamin C is somewhat acidic (like carbonated soft drinks), I recommend rinsing the mouth and teeth with water after taking it. Give your infant a chaser of plain water after he or she takes vitamin C from a dropper or spoon. If you are sensitive to acidity, you can also buy buffered vitamin C powder, such as calcium ascorbate, or nonacidic sodium ascorbate, or use nonacidic chewables. All these forms of vitamin C are available at health food stores or through the Internet. (I do not make brand recommendations.)

Hint 2: *Dose depends on need.* The sicker the child, the higher the dose. To learn more about this, you will definitely want to read the articles by Dr. Lendon Smith, Dr. Robert Cathcart, and Dr. Frederick Klenner, and books by Dr. Steve Hickey and Dr. Thomas Levy. See the back of the book for these references.

Hint 3: *Remember to put ALL the C in just SOME of the juice.* A child is more apt to down a small amount because it looks easy. My older brother tried to teach me how to ride a bicycle by putting me on his. It did not work, because I was afraid of being up too high. At a playground one day, I borrowed a little kid's tiny two-wheeler, and taught myself to ride it in five minutes. Later, I could ride my brother's big bike just fine.

Hint 4: *Use a sweet "chaser" drink to kill the sour taste.* Put all the C in a small volume of sweetened liquid, and after it's gone down the hatch, *immediately* have on hand a "chaser" of sweet, sweet juice. Reward their taste buds for bravely taking their C powder, and by golly they will keep doing it. For especially tricky kids, offering a tasty dessert food (such as a mouthful of ice cream or a big bite of cake) for a chaser makes it a lot less likely to come back up at you. Your children will correctly see this as the bribe it is. Just a spoonful of pastry helps the vitamins go down . . . and stay down.

Hint 5: *Think big, even in little people.* Remember: It takes a huge amount of vitamin C to act as an antiviral, antibiotic, antitoxin, or antihistamine. *Expect to have to use as much as 1,000 milligrams of vitamin C per pound of baby.* You may very well get a cure with less, but not a lot less. What works is what works.

Hint 6: *Get informed.* Do yourself and your children a favor and consult the following helpful resources. Both are available in their entirety, for free, on the Internet.

Dr. Klenner's *Clinical Guide to the Use of Vitamin C,* http://www.whale.to/a/smith_b .html

Irwin Stone's book *The Healing Factor,* at http://vitamincfoundation.org/stone/

Hint 7: *You can either use enough, or have a sick kid.* I made my decision nearly thirty years ago. My children were raised all the way into college without ever having had a singe dose of any antiviral or antibiotic. Of course they got sick sometimes. But it's how they got well that counts: We used vitamin C, and plenty of it.

Hint 8: *Buffer to reduce acidity.* To comfort especially sensitive tummies, buffer any excess acidity with any combination of calcium, food, and liquid. You can also buy nonacidic vitamin C (see Hint 1). This is especially tooth-friendly, and essential when purchasing chewables. Whether it's chewables or powder, nonacidic or not, get the child in the habit of rinsing their mouth with water after each dose. Vitamin C is about as acidic as a cola soft drink. Rinse after either one. Of course, like nose blowing, only the older toddler may get the hang of the art of rinsing.

Hint 9 (The Biggest Hint of All): *Bowel tolerance indicates saturation of vitamin C.* When junior is on the pot, the coughing and sneezing will be gone. See for yourself. This cannot be overemphasized. It's the number-one vitamin C therapy question that parents ask.

Is Your Child Healthier than a Lab Animal?

The United States RDA for vitamin C for humans is less than one-sixth of the government's vitamin C standard for guinea pigs. Why guinea pigs? We primates, guinea pigs, and fruit bats have a unique relationship. We have lost the ability to synthesize from glucose, on demand, the vitamin C our bodies need. Wait a minute; that cannot possibly be true. Can it?

The U.S. Department of Agriculture states that "the guinea pig's vitamin C requirement is 10–15 mg per day under normal conditions and 15–25 mg per day if pregnant, lactating, or growing."[6] That sounds reasonable. But how much is that compared to humans?

An adult guinea pig weighs about one kilogram (2.2 pounds). Guinea pigs therefore need between 10 and 25 milligrams of C per kilogram. In the Unite States, an average human weighs (at least) 82 kg (180 lbs).[7] An average three-year-old child weighs a tad over 13 kg, about 30 pounds. That means the USDA's standards, if applied to adults, would set our vitamin C requirement somewhere between 820 mg and 2,000 mg vitamin C per day. If fairly applied to growing children, the vitamin C RDA for a three-year-old would be between 90 and 150 mg.

The official U.S. RDAs for vitamin C are different than these. Quite different. They are lower. Much lower.

The U.S. RDA per day for vitamin C for adult humans is 90 mg for men; 75 mg for women. For smokers, they allow an additional 35 mg. For children one to three years old, the RDA is a mere 15 mg. If your three-year old were a guinea pig, he or she would be getting six to ten times more than that.

Why are we humans repeatedly urged to consume only the RDA when the RDA is considerably less of the government's official nutrient requirement for an animal?

THE COST OF KIDS' VITAMINS BUGGING YOU?

Oh, please. The average baby goes through between 6,000 and 7,000 diapers before completing toilet training. You might just as well have a healthy baby as a dry baby. (We mentioned this in the Feeding chapter, but it bears repeating!)

Reminder to all out readers: We do not have any financial connection to the health products industry. We do not endorse any supplement brand, and we do not provide recommendations as to which one you might want to use. That is what Google searches and health food stores are for.

WHEN EVIDENCE IS A CHOICE

"High dosage of vitamin C for little children? If it were so good, my pediatrician would already know about it. Where is the evidence?"

A few years ago, Dr. Abram Hoffer said to me, "Perhaps you should write a tongue-in-cheek paper, in which you announce, "Antibiotics Do Not Cure Infection." Then, somewhere hidden in the paper, report that you only gave 200 units or even 20,000 units of a drug that requires doses of one million or more."

As always, Dr. Hoffer set my mind in motion, and this is the result.

It is a cornerstone of medical science that dose affects treatment outcome. This premise is accepted in pharmaceutical drug therapy, but not with nutrient therapy. In nutritional therapy, dose is also very important. That hardly seems a provocative statement, but it is. High doses were advocated almost immediately after ascorbic acid was isolated by Albert Szent-Gyorgyi, M.D. (1893–1986). Notable early medical pioneers of high-dose vitamin C (ascorbate) therapy are Claus Washington Jungeblut, M.D. (1898–1976); William J. McCormick, M.D. (1880–1968); and Frederick R. Klenner, M.D. (1907–1984). More recently, important work has been published by Hugh D. Riordan, M.D. (1932–2005) and Robert F. Cathcart III, M.D. (1932–2007). Drs. Evan and Wilfrid Shute said the same about vitamin E, and Dr. Hoffer spoke similarly about niacin.

Investigators using nutrients in high doses have consistently reported success. Dr. Frederick Robert Klenner wrote, "If you want results, use adequate ascorbic acid."[8] The medical literature has ignored such "anecdotal" physician reports and nearly eighty years of controlled (but not double-blind-placebo-controlled) clinical studies on high-dose nutrient therapy.

Evidence-based anything is only as good as the evidence collected. You can set up any experiment to fail. One way to ensure failure is to create a meaningless test. A meaningless test is guaranteed, if you use insufficient quantities of the substance to be investigated. Randomized controlled trials (RCTs) of high vitamin doses are very rare. RCTs with low doses of nutrients are plentiful. Low doses don't work. Performing a meta-analysis of many low-dose studies teaches nothing worth knowing. The first rule of building a brick wall is that you have to have enough bricks.

Some twenty years ago, Robert F. Cathcart, M.D., wrote:

> As evidence of the value of nutrients, especially vitamin C . . . becomes more and more evident to the public, researchers produce a mass of articles on minute aspects of vitamin C. I have been consulted by many researchers who proposed bold studies of the effects of massive doses of ascorbate. Every time the university center, the ethics committee, the pharmacy committee, etc. deny permission for the use of massive doses of ascorbate and render the study almost useless. Seasoned researchers depending upon government grants do not even try to study adequate doses. All of this results in a massive accumulation of knowledge about very little which gives the impression that there is no more of real importance to be learned. This accumulation of minutia hides the great effects of ascorbate already known by some. . . . As you read these learned papers, you will realize that they seem to be completely unaware of the uses of massive doses of ascorbate. One of the most amusing aspects of this research are the speculations and research into the toxicity and other adverse reactions of tiny doses of ascorbate when many have used for years 20 to 100 times the amounts being discussed.[9]

Dosage is set by the researcher. In terms of experimental design, it is not much harder to use 2,000 milligrams than to use 200 mg. Effective doses are high doses, often 1,000 times more than the U.S. RDA or Daily Reference Intake (DRI). Most unsuccessful vitamin C research has used inadequate, low doses. Low doses do not get clinical results. Investigators may choose to test only low nutrient doses because of arbitrary "safe upper limits." Such limits, largely theoretical, effectively keep Institutional Review Boards (IRSs) from allowing megadose research. I have colleagues who serve on IRBs. None of them knew that, in the entire United States, there was not even one death caused by a dietary supplement in 2008.[10] Zero reported deaths from vitamins, minerals, herbs and amino acids does not mean that they are unconditionally safe. It does, however, strongly suggest that nutrients in large doses are safer than pharmaceuticals in any dose. A good case could be made that nutrient "safe upper limits" are themselves not evidence based.

Investigators may choose to employ low-nutrient doses because they are unaware, or choose to be unaware, of established high-dose benefits. Or, investigators may claim that they are in fact using high doses, and editorialize as such in their conclusions. Linus Pauling specifically warned against this in his first orthomolecular book, *Vitamin C and the Common Cold*. Forty years later, we still see new nutritional research presenting 500 mg or 1,000 mg of ascorbate as if these were a lot. With a safe upper limit dictated at 2,000 mg, where is the surprise?

What constitutes evidence? The majority of medical interventions have never been rigorously tested. A mere 11 percent have been shown to be beneficial, and another 23 percent are "likely to be beneficial."[11] Conventional chemotherapy for cancer contributes only 2.3 percent to five-year cancer survival in Australia and 2.1 percent in the United States.[12] It would be difficult to make a case that such treatment is evidence based. Indeed, many an oncologist will recommend chemotherapy for patients with a cancer against which chemo is known to be ineffective.

If you think medical research may allow for some flexible truth, you should consider nutrition, and the guinea pig example given above.

Shooting beans at a charging rhinoceros is not likely to influence the outcome. If you were to give every homeless person you met on the street twenty-five cents, you could easily prove that money will not help poverty. The public and their doctors look to scientific researchers to test and confirm the efficacy of any nutritional therapy. As long as such research that is done uses small doses of vitamins, doses that are too small to work, orthomolecular medicine will be touted as "unproven." Things are looking up with more and more published high-dose vitamin D research. Now we'll have to wait for the rest of the alphabet.

PLANNING TO HAVE MORE CHILDREN?

Okay, maybe your young 'un is still in diapers and barely sleeping through the night. Still, one-child families are the exception, not the rule. So, thinking (and mutually discussing and, we sincerely hope, planning) ahead, consider the following:

A randomized, double-blind, placebo-controlled fourteen-day trial of 3,000 mg per day of vitamin C reported that there was greater frequency of sexual intercourse in the vitamin C group (but not the placebo group). The vitamin C group also experienced a decrease in Beck Depression scores.

The authors said that this effect is probably due to the fact that vitamin C "modulates catecholaminergic activity, decreases stress reactivity, approach anxiety and prolactin release, improves vascular function, and increases oxytocin release. These processes are relevant to sexual behavior and mood."[1]

At any rate, it is a little something extra about vitamin C that you might find worth knowing. Also, remember the stand-up comic's newsflash that the cause of sibling rivalry has now been discovered. It is having more than one child. Birth control is valuable . . . especially if you are going to try your own confirmation of the above study.

Reference

1. Brody, S. "High-Dose Ascorbic Acid Increases Intercourse Frequency and Improves Mood: A Randomized Controlled Clinical Trial." *Biol Psychiatry* 52(4) Aug 15, 2002):371–374.

VITAMIN SUPPLEMENTS FOR NUTRITIONALLY DEPRIVED CHILDREN

Vitamin C has been proven to have striking beneficial effect on the health of children with chronic nutritional insufficiency. Vitamin C has become part of the daily lives of the Myky tribe in Brazil's Goias rainforests, thanks to the efforts of Sister Suzie Wills and a number of other Sisters of St. Joseph. Sr. Wills has been very effective in getting native people not only eating citrus fruits and berries but also taking

C powder and tablets on a regular basis. She reports healthier children and babies, and that infant mortality has dramatically decreased.

A reader writes:

> My husband and I adopted a fifteen-month old boy from China in March, 2002. He was tiny for his age, had rickets and bald spots, and brittle hair. We began supplementing immediately with liquid vitamins. Since then, with good nutrition and TLC, he's made huge improvements. But as of January, 2003, he still had not attained the lowest percentile on the U.S. weight charts. He's always been a very big eater, especially for a toddler; the doc calls this "compensatory eating." After a conversation within our family about how to help the little guy put on some more weight, and research (including your newsletter and site), I began giving him vitamin C. We worked our way up to 3 grams a day and about one-eighth of a tablet of 100 mg niacin for toddler temper, as needed.
>
> At his next weight check in April, the fellow had put on two and a half pounds, thus edging his way onto the weight charts. The doc was very impressed. I believe the addition of the vitamin C really helped him put a little weight on his bones. He stayed remarkably healthy. The doc remarked that he was expecting to see him for flu, winter colds, or at least something, given his somewhat compromised nutritional status. I also think the vitamin C helped him fight off colds. He is in a preschool, and has come home with sniffles, but at the first sign I would aggressively supplement with C and he'd gobble them down: up to 12,000 milligrams for a twenty-five pound boy with no diarrhea. It really works.

THE SAFETY OF VITAMIN C

"There has to be a safety issue in here somewhere."

That's many a reader's first concern when presented with the idea of enormous vitamin C doses. And you're right. There is indeed a safety issue, and here it is: *Vitamin C (ascorbic acid) is safer than any medication on the market. Period.*

ARTHUR M. SACKLER, M.D. (1913–1987)
Orthomolecular Medicine Hall of Fame 2006

Arthur Sackler, M.D., the famous philanthropist, physician, and publisher of the highly respected *Medical Tribune* newspaper, was born in Brooklyn and educated at New York University. He worked at Lincoln Hospital in New York City as an intern and house physician and completed his residency in psychiatry at Creedmoor State Hospital. His National Academies of Sciences biography states that "there, in the 1940s, he started research that resulted in more than 150 papers in neuroendocrinology, psychiatry, and experimental medicine."

Dr. Sackler started the *Medical Tribune* in 1960. It would grow to an international readership of over one million, with Sackler himself contributing over 500 articles on a wide variety of health issues. In 1981, Sackler ran a page-one story on Ruth Harrell's study showing that high doses of vitamins improve IQ in Down syndrome children. In one 1982 column, he personally declared his support for bowel-tolerance doses of ascorbate, including with his comments the text of "a letter we just received from Robert Cathcart III, M.D. "whom Sackler described as "brilliant." Many physicians first saw these words in the *Tribune*: "Ascorbic acid administered orally to bowel tolerance (just short of producing diarrhea) has a definite antipyretic effect [and] administered IM [intramuscular] to small infants will usually have a dramatic effect on elevated temperatures."

The most common side effect of vitamin C is failure to take enough of it. The other common side effects are loose stools (which are a marker of saturation) and upset stomach, usually due to lack of buffering. Buffering means reducing vitamin C's acidity by taking it with a meal, snack, beverage, calcium tablet, or by using a nonacidic form. This is discussed more fully in Steve Hickey and Andrew Saul's *Vitamin C: The Real Story*.

"My doctor doesn't believe in vitamins."

Since when is medicine based on belief?

Heard this one before? "If vitamin C was that good, doctors would tell their patients to take a lot of it." It is surprising how many physicians are doing precisely that. What's that? Your doctor still doesn't? Why? Decades of physicians' reports and controlled studies support the use of very large doses of vitamin C. The medical literature has virtually ignored seventy-five years of physician reports and laboratory and clinical studies on successful high-dose vitamin C therapy.

VITAMIN C, INFECTIOUS DISEASES, AND TOXINS: CURING THE INCURABLE

Thomas E. Levy, a practicing physician for twenty-five years, is a board-certified internist and a fellow of the American College of Cardiology. He is also an attorney. What's more, he's a really fine writer. Dr. Levy's book, *Vitamin C, Infectious Diseases, and Toxins: Curing the Incurable* immediately made my most select list of absolutely required reading. That list is rather short.

The key figure in vitamin C research, chest specialist and ascorbic acid megadose pioneer Frederick R. Klenner, M.D. is usually omitted entirely from most orthodox nutrition, health, or medical texts. The importance of Klenner's clinical observations showing vitamin C's power against infectious and chronic disease is extraordinary. Dr. Levy intends that you become familiar with Klenner's work, and *Vitamin C, Infectious Diseases, and Toxins* accomplishes this purpose with distinction.

"It is completely appropriate to use the term "cure" when, in fact, the evidence demonstrates that a given medical condition has clearly and repeatedly been cured by a specific therapy . . . Avoiding the use of a term such as "cure" when it is absolutely appropriate does as much harm as using it inappropriately. Not realizing the incredible ability of vitamin C to cure a given infectious disease just perpetuates the usage of so many other needlessly applied toxic drugs and clinical protocols. If the shoe fits, wear it, and if the treatment works, proclaim it." (p 15)

And this is precisely what Dr. Levy does.

"Properly dosed vitamin C will reliably and quickly cure nearly all cases of acute polio and acute hepatitis. Polio babies are completely well in less than a week and hepatitis patients are sick for only a few days, not several months." (p 19)

Knowing full well how the medical profession will react to such statements, Dr. Levy writes: "Unquestioning faith in the "established" medical knowledge is so deeply ingrained that many doctors simply will not even consider reading something that comes from sources that they do not consider worthy of producing new medical concepts. And if they do . . . they quickly dismiss it as just being ridiculous if it conflicts with too many of the concepts that most of their colleagues and textbooks embrace." (p 22)

Aside from personally conducing their own mostly pre-Medline journal search, the primary way patients (and through them, their physicians) have been exposed to Dr. Klenner's work has been through Lendon Smith's sixty-eight-page *Clinical Guide to the Use of Vitamin C: The Clinical Experiences of Frederick R. Klenner, M.D.*

My college students' avoidance response when I trot out "old" megavitamin studies is nothing compared to the sheer hostility I have received from academic colleagues. Once one of my undergraduates submitted a paper in another class discussing some twenty fairly old medical references she had found on vitamin C as a cure for polio. That course's instructor told me privately that the student's work was absurd, and he literally described her as a "dial tone." I recall a nutritional presentation I made to a hospital staff. All was going well until I mentioned using vitamin C as an antibiotic, as Dr. Klenner did. The mood changed quickly.

Acceptance is not helped by the fact that most of Dr. Klenner's papers were published between twenty-five and fifty-five years ago. Says Dr. Levy: "Many physicians have outright disdain for any medical literature that is more than a few years old. It almost seems that even the best scientific data is considered to have a "shelf life," and . . . will never be appreciated unless a "modern" researcher decides to repeat the study and "rediscover" the information." (p 27)

And when such modern "reproductions" are done, they commonly use far too little vitamin C: "I could find no mainstream medical researcher who has performed *any* clinical studies on *any* infectious disease with vitamin C does that approached those used by Klenner. Using a small enough dose of any therapeutic agent will demonstrate little or no effect on an infection or disease process. Klenner would often use daily doses of vitamin C on a patient that would be as much as 10,000 times more than the daily doses used in some of the many clinical studies in the literature." (p 28–29)

Because there are few families that will not be affected by serious infectious illness, the individual topics Dr. Levy addresses (in Chapter 2, constituting 130 pages) are especially important. These include measles, mumps, viral encephalitis, herpes, mononucleosis, viral pneumonia, chicken pox, Ebola, and of course influenza. He has included a fairly lengthy section on acquired immune deficiency syndrome (AIDS). Rabies is an intriguing entry, even to those already willing to concede that vitamin C is an effective antiviral.

Here is an example of vitamin C therapy for mononucleosis:

Vitamin C proved to be useful when my five-year-old contracted it (proved by a blood test). His fever spiked to 104.3 overnight and his glands swelled like chipmunk cheeks. A visit to the pediatrician came with a warning that he'd likely be down for a week or more. Three days of megadose C and he was tearing around with the neighbor kids and back to his usual smart-alecky self.

I knew what the answer would be when I asked the M.D. about treatments for mono, but I just smiled quietly to myself and suppressed a laugh when Dr. There's-Nothing-You-Can-Do-for-a-Virus answered with a flippant "rest, fluids, kiddie Tylenol" as I knew he would. What matters is that we know what to do when the viral train rolls through: reach for the "C" and take plenty.

Nonviral diseases discussed include diphtheria, tuberculosis (in considerable detail), strep, brucellosis, typhoid, dysentery, malaria, trichinosis, and the always-controversial subjects of tetanus and pertussis. Not unexpectedly, Dr. Levy seems to incline towards the nontraditional viewpoint on vaccination, although since the book lacks an index, his statements on this specific subject take a moment to locate. As vitamin C is such a good antibiotic and antiviral, a de-emphasis on vaccination can be seen to make sense.

Ascorbic acid, that Swiss Army knife among nutrients, has been unjustly dismissed in part because of the implausibility of such very great utility. A human body of tens of trillions of cells operates thousands of biochemical reactions on less than a dozen vitamins. Is it so very surprising that one nutrient would have so many benefits?

"The Ultimate Antidote" (Chapter 3, 103 pages) considers vitamin C as an antitoxin. This chapter will, as Mark Twain put it, gratify some and astonish the rest. The effects of alcohol, the barbiturates, carbon monoxide, cyanide, aflatoxin, a variety of environmental poisons including pesticides, even acetaminophen poisoning in cats, mushroom poisoning, and snake venoms are all shown to respond to vitamin C megadose therapy. Mercury, lead, and the effects of radiation receive special and really eye-opening attention.

If there is a greater calling than healing the sick, it is teaching people how to do it themselves. Abram Hoffer and Lendon H. Smith are perhaps the two foremost examples of physician-authors who have focused on directly instructing their readers how to use megavitamins correctly and directly. I think Dr. Levy is another of these natural-born teachers, and this may be most apparent in the book's section of "Practical Suggestions" (Chapter 5). General readers, having just learned that high oral doses of ascorbate are effective for self-medication, will appreciate receiving the benefits of Dr. Levy's professional experience. Physician readers will especially welcome his injection instructions. I would like to see this important chapter greatly expanded.

A book this good deserves a more eye-catching, upscale cover to attract bookshelf attention and get to those who most need it. I hope the next edition will also add some visual aids. Opponents to medical use of vitamin C will almost certainly demand expansion of Chapter 4 ("The Safety of High Doses of Vitamin C") to include more negative studies and more commentary on possible negative effects of massive doses of ascorbate. Dr. Levy does in fact devote considerable attention to hemochromatosis, immune system concerns, G6PD deficiency, allegations of DNA damage and kidney stone formation, the rebound effect, and vitamin C's pro-oxidant characteristics. I doubt if any chapter of any length would satisfy vitamin therapy's harshest critics. Furthermore, they can always find abundant (if mostly unfounded) ammunition in practically any medical or nutrition textbook in print. In Levy's book, there is a welcome emphasis on the positive side of vitamin C megadoses, and that is their power to cure the sick.

There is no doubt whatsoever that Dr. Klenner would wholeheartedly approve of Dr. Levy stating this (p 36): "The three most important considerations in effective vitamin C therapy are "dose, dose, and dose. If you don't take enough, you won't get the desired effects. Period!"

Dr. Levy's book presents clear evidence that vitamin C cures disease. It contains over 1,200 scientific references, presented chapter by chapter. It does not mince words. It is disease specific. It is dose specific. It is practical. It is readable. It is excellent.

This review was originally was published in the *Journal of Orthomolecular Medicine,* Vol. 18, No. 2, 2003, p 117–118. It is reprinted here (with some revision) with permission.

INTRAVENOUS VITAMIN C FIGHTS TETANUS

"The effect of daily *intravenous* administration of 1,000 mg ascorbic acid (AA, vitamin C) in tetanus patients aged 1–30 years was studied. In the age group of 1–12 years, 31 patients were treated with AA as additional to antitetanus serum, sedatives and antibiotics. It was found that *none of the patients died who received AA* along with the conventional antitetanus therapy. On the other hand, 74.2 percent of the tetanus patients who received the conventional antitetanus therapy without AA (control group) were succumbed to the infection." (My emphasis.)

Look at that nearly thirty-year old paper again, and wince: Three-quarters of kids with tetanus died when treated with conventional medication. Yet a mere 1,000 mg/day of injected vitamin C was enough to save all of those to whom it was given.

Reference

Jahan, K., K. Ahmad, M. A. Ali. "Effect of Ascorbic Acid in the Treatment of Tetanus." *Bangladesh Med Res Counc Bull* 10(1) (Jun 1984):24–28.

Whatever Happened to Vitamin C Therapy for Polio?

Dr. Jungeblut, Professor of Bacteriology at Columbia University, first published about vitamin C as prevention and treatment for polio in 1935.[1] Jungeblut used fairly low doses. Albert Sabin used even lower doses, normally only one-third of Jungeblut's. Sabin's unsuccessful "replication" was taken as the definitive standard, and remains ineffectively so to this day. Even with relatively low doses of vitamin C, Jungeblut made the correct conclusions.

Also in 1935, Jungeblut showed that vitamin C inactivated the diphtheria toxin.[2] By 1937, Jungeblut demonstrated that ascorbate inactivated tetanus toxin.[3] Between 1943 and 1947, Dr. Klenner, a specialist in diseases of the chest, cured forty-one cases of viral pneumonia with vitamin C. By 1946, Dr. McCormick showed how vitamin C prevents and also cures kidney stones; by 1957, how it fights cardiovascular disease. Beginning in the 1960s, Dr. Cathcart used large doses of vitamin C to treat pneumonia, hepatitis, and eventually AIDS. For more than three decades, beginning in 1975, Dr. Riordan and his team have successfully used large doses of intravenous vitamin C against cancer. The use of doses of tens of thousands of milligrams of vitamin C per day may be the most unacknowledged successful research in medicine.

BUT *POLIO*?

"When I first came across Klenner's work on polio patients," writes cardiologist and attorney Dr. Thomas Levy, "I was absolutely amazed and even a bit overwhelmed at what I read . . . To know that polio had been easily cured and so many babies, children, and some adults still continued to die or survive to be permanently crippled by this virus was extremely difficult to accept. . . . Even more incredibly, Klenner briefly presented a summarization of his work on polio at the Annual Session of the American Medical Association on June 10, 1949, in Atlantic City, New Jersey:

> It might be interesting to learn how poliomyelitis was treated in Reidsville, N.C., during the 1948 epidemic. In the past seven years, virus infections have been treated and cured in a period of seventy-two hours by the employment of massive frequent injections of ascorbic acid, or vitamin C. I believe that if vitamin C in these massive doses—6,000 to 20,000 mg in a twenty-four hour period—is given to these patients with poliomyelitis none will be paralyzed and there will be no further maiming or epidemics of poliomyelitis.

"The four doctors who commented after Klenner did not have anything to say about his assertions."[4]

Check the Recommended Reading section at the end of this book for more resources and information about these authors.

References

1. Jungeblut, C. W. "Inactivation of Poliomyelitis Virus in vitro by Crystalline Vitamin C (Ascorbic Acid)." *J Exper Med* 62(4) (Sep 30, 1935):517–521.

2. Jungeblut, C. W., R. L. Zwemer. "Inactivation of Diphtheria Toxin in vivo and in vitro by Crystalline Vitamin C (Ascorbic Acid)." *Proc Soc Exper Biol Med* 32(8) (May 1935):1229–1234.

3. Jungeblut, C. W. "Inactivation of Tetanus Toxin by Crystalline Vitamin C (l-Ascorbic Acid). *J Immunol* 33(3) (Sep 1, 1937):203–214.

4. Levy, T. E. *Vitamin C, Infectious Diseases, and Toxins: Curing the Incurable.* Philadelphia, PA: Xlibris Corporation, 2002.

Bias Against Ascorbate Therapy

When you pick up a health or nutrition book and want to know really fast if it is any good or not, just check the index for "Klenner" and three other key names: Cathcart, Stone, and Pauling. Robert F. Cathcart, an orthopedic surgeon, administered huge doses of vitamin C to tens of thousands of patients for decades,[13] without generating a single kidney stone. If a book has negative things to say about Linus Pauling, you are not likely to find a fair hearing for vitamins. Irwin Stone, the biochemist who first put Linus Pauling onto vitamin C, is the author of *The Healing Factor: Vitamin C Against Disease.*[14] Pauling cites Stone thirteen times in his landmark book *How to Live Longer and Feel Better,*[15] a recommendation if there ever was one. The importance of vitamin C's power against infectious and chronic disease is extraordinary. To me, omitting it is tantamount to deleting Shakespeare from an English Lit course.

Cardiologist Thomas Levy, M.D., explains: "I could find no mainstream medical researcher who has performed any clinical studies on any infectious disease with vitamin C doses that approached those used by Klenner. Using a small enough dose of any therapeutic agent will demonstrate little or no effect on an infection or disease process."[17]

It is high time for medical professionals to welcome vitamin C megadoses and their power to cure the sick. Cure is by far the best word there is in medicine. It would seem that you cannot spell "cure" without "C." I do not think Dr. Klenner would dispute that.

CHAPTER 15

ENVIRONMENTAL HAZARDS AFFECTING INFANTS AND TODDLERS

Parents are bombarded with one-sided, upsetting information presented on television and in popular magazines. That is why I (RKC) feel strongly that we have to set the record straight. We've explained the detoxifying effect of vitamin C and the value of good nutrition and vitamin supplements in this book, but you should also be aware of the "toxifying" chemicals we encounter in our day-to-day lives, and how to protect yourself and your children from them. Also, keep in mind that the media likes to revive "shocking" safety issues when there are no current "breakthrough" studies. Recently, we were alarmed to hear of arsenic in rice. This was studied eight years earlier, at which time it was determined that inorganic arsenic, not organic, was the culprit. Inorganic arsenic has been used as a pesticide—a practice that has been banned for years. Naturally occurring organic forms of arsenic are relatively harmless. Attention to specific pollutants comes and goes. Radon gas, which occurs naturally in the earth, can seep into a house from the basement or through the floor. It is a radioactive material, and it was a truly "hot" item of concern in the 1980s and on, for several years. Radon is a decay product of uranium, and its own decay products can take the form of dust. The half-life of the gas is short (3.8 days) and would be of little significance except in areas of poor air exchange, as in a deep mine or an airtight, energy-efficient building. It can also be found in higher concentrations in the water from hot springs. One would think that an environmental problem associated with the word "uranium" would not fade away, but much less attention is paid towards radon today. (Associate the words "uranium" and "Iran" and we create many lively discussions.)

With industrialization comes pollution. Let me describe a few pollutants that are deemed newsworthy. (It should be pointed out at the beginning that no matter how long we have known about a chemical's toxicity, media attention often seems to enjoy presenting an old scare in a new format.) The following are the primary offenders that you've probably heard of, and that we need to watch out for.

We need to keep in mind that detoxifying takes place in the liver. In the young child, and especially in the infant, the immature liver does not work at full capacity. They, and the unborn, need special consideration.

THE INFAMOUS HEAVY METALS

Lead may have the record of being the "show," with the longest-running attention-getting news articles, with mercury not far behind. New angles of their dangers are continuously reported.

Mercury

The silver liquid elemental mercury, is relatively harmless unless it is vaporized. The real culprits are the organic forms—methyl and ethyl mercury. The Minamata incident, which involved mercury, was probably one of the most egregious environmental disasters ever known. Minamata is a small factory town on Minamata Bay in Japan's westernmost island. In 1956 many cases of infantile cerebral palsy (spastic paralysis) began turning up. It seemed improbable that after witnessing just a few of these twisted, terribly damaged infants, that little was done to determine the cause. Eventually, it was determined that *methyl* mercury was the culprit. Since 1932, mercury in one form or the other was being discharged into the bay from the local chemical plant. The discharge may have been elemental mercury originally, but through interaction with bacterial and other organic material inherent to the water over the years, it gradually transformed to methyl mercury.

Ethyl mercury had its use many years ago in the form of Merthiolate (better known by its trade name Mercurochrome), a red solution that was painted on even minor cuts or abrasions to kill nasty germs. There was great faith in its powers, so that it was occasionally even painted on infected tonsils with a cotton-tipped swab, causing all sorts of uncontrolled gagging in child victims. Ethyl mercury is still found as a component of thimerosal, which is used as a preservative in some vaccines. It came to the public's attention after Dr. Andrew Wakefield's 1998 publication that linked autism to the MMR (mumps, measles, rubella) vaccine. He felt that the main issue was that the measles virus adversely influenced the immune system, as evidenced by abnormalities in the intestinal lymphoid system and the nervous system. He advocated giving the three components of the MMR separately.

The "war" began. All sorts of weak studies poured in, allegedly reporting to link the MMR vaccine, preserved with thimerosal, to autism. Many parents became concerned that the use of the vaccine would lead to autism, and refused vaccination for their children. Vaccination producers felt threatened. A "gold-standard" theory-bashing study was performed in Denmark (why not in the U.S.?) that claimed to put an end to the "autism-MMR link" theory. A closer look revealed a poorly designed study that proved nothing. Diligent fact-finding studies were conducted, including a Senate Investigating Committee report emphasizing that the safe levels for mercury in the immature nervous system were set too high. The FDA was stimulated to review its "safe" levels and imposed regulations that reduced the amount of thimerosal in vaccines and the number of thimerosal-containing vaccines.

In 1999 (within a year after the Danish paper was published) the Academy of Pediatrics Handbook for pediatricians announced, "Because some infants who receive thimerosal-containing vaccines during the early months of life *could* be exposed to more mercury than recommended by Federal guidelines, in July of 1999 the U.S. government *asked* manufacturers to eliminate *or reduce, expeditiously as possible,* the mercury content of their vaccines." (My emphasis.) How's that for taking a tough stance? "Expeditiously as possible" proved to translate as, "We will make as little change as we can get away with." There has been *some,* but not complete, improvement in lowering thimerosal content in vaccines. A study that measured mercury levels in immunized infants versus levels in nonvaccinated infants showed that the immunized have *levels of mercury within the FDA standard of safety*. There is the rub. What are safe standards? The Standards are revised only whenever there is enough pressure from those concerned about health effects to motivate change. It is fair to ask your shot-giver to inform you of the thimerosal content of the vaccines he or she is administering. Pestering may get results.

The Wakefield issue is muddied by finding that the author of a piece published in British medical journals that claimed that Dr. Wakefield had altered his data had ties to the vaccine industry himself. So now the courts will attempt to determine what is right.

Mercury by land and by sea. How about by air? It is tough for me to visualize, but mercury vapor from coal-fired electrical plants in China can make its way to our shores in amounts that make environmental experts nervous. Couple this with acid rain produced from fossil fuel burning and we have a double-whammy effect on the diet of fish in affected waters. A newly created mercury vapor hazard is present when an energy-efficient light bulb is broken. The safety warning for cleanup of a broken bulb is quite extensive—almost scary.

Later on, we will tell you how to survive this toxic world. Things aren't as bad as they are portrayed. As for saving energy by introducing an energy-efficient bulb to replace the incandescent light bulb, I wonder if our legislators thought about the best saving device of all—the light switch? The best gas saver is the ignition switch. There are no emissions problems associated with the use of these gadgets.

Lead

Lead has a sordid history. Thankfully, most of it *is* history. The impact on infant and children's health was very prominent before the use of tetraethyl lead in gasoline (added to prevent "knocking," or premature ignition) and lead in interior paints was stopped. For decades lead from gas engine exhaust was thrust into the air we breathed and dusted onto edible crops that were grown near highways. Old, inter-city housing had walls covered with peeling leaded paint. The children of the occupants would strip off the paint and eat it, due to a condition called "pica." Poor children with poor diets (and with parents poorly equipped to keep an eye on their children) develop strange cravings for trace minerals lacking in their diets. The best counter for this condition is vitamin C, a good all-around diet, and a watchful supervisor. Nutrition education and provision of vitamin C-containing foods would go a long ways toward solving the problem, but this solution would be slow to take effect. So leaded paints and ethyl gasoline were banned, and landlords were *encouraged* (not required) to scrape the walls of their rental units.

Lead toxicity should not be taken lightly, as it has a drastic effect on the blood-forming system and the brain, especially of the young. The big pollution factors have been successfully dealt with. Undue fear of poisoning should cease. All that is left are concern about little ones ingesting lead-coated toys or trinkets that illegally enter our market place. There was a time when a great furor was generated by imports from China. Fortunately, our government brought these imports to a halt. I didn't feel as much concern, because I could not fathom how a toddler could dismantle a toy, swallow whole big junks of it, or chew it, with only a maximum of one two-year-old molar in each quadrant of his or her mouth.

CHEMICAL SOUP

We are stuck with a diet of chemical soup. As with any soup, we should know the ingredients—so we can add more good ingredients and get rid of the bad as much as possible. If a chemical or a natural element such as arsenic is found in our food or water, we should pay attention to tests for carcinogenicity (cancer causing) in man or beast, and do our best to determine "safe" levels—in other words, what is tolerable by the body, and, also, what can be readily countered with nutrition.

A negative spin-off of new "energy-efficient buildings" was the finding that many pollutants can be trapped inside the building when there is inadequate fresh air turnover. My personal experience as a Health Officer was finding that school personnel were getting sicker through the week and recuperating, somewhat, over the weekend. Formaldehyde in new carpet backing was the cause of this "sick building syndrome." This problem, too, was remedied. The remedy includes making the building "leak" enough air to turn the air over every three hours. New building codes have found a way to preserve efficiency without toxicity.

Bisphenol A

Bisphenol A has probably received the most bad press in the past few years of all of the unhealthy chemicals that have been introduced into our "better living" society. It is also called Bisphenol-A, or BPA.

BPAs have been removed from baby bottles at this point, and many companies are beginning to tout their "BPA-free" storage containers and adult drinking bottles. Interestingly, the Food and Drug Administration (FDA) had been under the gun to ban the use of BPA in baby bottles as other countries had done. Finally, in July of 2012, they did ban it, only to find that the industry had already voluntarily done so. The latest hullabaloo, however, is about BPA in the lining of food cans—a problem that had been dormant until the baby bottle and plastic container problem was solved.

The reason this has become a concern is that BPA is known to be a hormone disrupter that accumulate in fatty tissues. Putting two and two together—this factor and the rise in the number of obese kids in our society—research studies were performed, and BPA was found to be at higher levels in the urine samples of obese kids than in those of normal children.[1]

Polychlorinated Biphenyls (PCBs)

So, just what are PCBs, and how were they dispersed so that they got into our food chain? Wikipedia tells of the properties that make some of them useful for certain industrial applications. Mixed PCBs (there are several different kinds) are very stable and non-inflammable, have a high boiling point, and have a high electrical insulating effect. These properties make them suitable for use in transmitters and hydraulic fluids, to name a few prominent applications. They are very slow to break down—good for the industry; bad for the environment. Manufacturing sites are particularly contaminated by PCB spills because of this. Similar contamination occurs "in the field" from careless handling or leakage of the finished product. They are virtually insoluble in water. When they are released from industrial plants or other sources near bodies of water—coastal, river, or lake—they sink to the bottom and remain there, providing part of a poor diet for fish. So contamination in bodies of water varies with the industrial activity in the surrounds.

The affinity of PCBs for being stored in the fat of living creatures, and the idea of a food chain made up of little fish being eaten by bigger fish, brings us to the "good" fish—"bad" fish dilemma. "Cold water" (fatty) fish are a great source of the essential omega-3 fatty acids. (See the feeding chapter.) Unfortunately this health benefit can be somewhat countered by PCBs stored in the flesh of these fish, which feed in contaminated waters. It is hard for the FDA to set standards on safety because one body of water is not like another. One fish is not like another. The best they can come up with is an attempt to determine the maximum number and size of servings per week that would be safe for pregnant women and for children. They don't really have a database from different areas, which could vary from "relatively pure" to "toxic." The problem is made more complex if these same sources have contamination from mercury or other chemicals. So it is difficult for authorities like the American Academy of Pediatrics (AAP) to make definite recommendations. The best bet is to check the source of the fish you eat and determine your own estimate of safety. I suggest that you pay more attention to the toxic effects when considering the diet of nursing or pregnant mothers and infants, and more to the beneficial effects when feeding children and grownups. The problem is not one, big toxic dose but long-term, small doses that accumulate in the body.

There are compounds in the group of chemicals we call PCBs that have properties similar to dioxins—the most potent chemical "bad guys" known to man. (Remember Agent Orange? It was a dioxin producer.) They are strong endocrine disrupters and have high neurotoxicity. The potential for causing birth defects is huge, making this a particularly important issue to consider for maternal, fetal, and infant health. The FDA recognizes their carcinogenicity and has put a maximum "safe" level at 0.5 parts per million (ppm).

The limited industrial use of PCBs initially had greatly expanded after a few years, as it found its way into transformers and capacitors and things as diversified as fire-retardant fibers. This latter application translated to fire-retardant-treated pajamas for children. When the toxicity of PCB was documented, the practice of surrounding our children with such things as "safe" pajamas—without real studies of safety—created an outrage, and led to a ban in 1973 on using BPAs for this purpose. It was not anticipated that transformers and capacitors would leak, or could catch fire (the containers, themselves), or explode, releasing large amounts of toxic materials into the environment. Such events accounted for a small percentage of spills, but they quickly became a small percentage of a huge number. Industrial use in new equipment was banned in 1981. Existing equipment was grandfathered in, under the regulations, until December, 2000. At this point PCBs persistence in the environment is been the problem, much like the situation after the pesticide DDT was banned.

Environmental detectives throughout the industrial world found that there was serious PCB contamination in chicken feed, beef, and drinking water. And as we have seen with other contaminants, health issues were well known by some manufacturers, but corporate decisions were based on what they could get away with. Which would cost more: paying an Environmental Protection Agency (EPA) fine or going to the expense of compliance with the regulations? Some pretty sleazy cover-ups took place as a result. Way back in the 1940s, one company gave away "guaranteed clean" soil that came from an EPA cleanup site to get the EPA off its back. The company executives were fully aware that the soil was distinctly *un*clean. In North Carolina, in 1978, masked drivers in black trucks dumped their cleanup material along the shoulders of the highway in the black of night. (These horror stories are described in Wikipedia.)

Since EPA and FDA safety standards and regulations usually lag far behind the uncovering of new information, we can not wait for action on their part. We must continuously do our best to keep informed and keep our children safe and healthy. When big money is part of the equation, bad things happen. A bit of healthy skepticism is in order.

Perchlorate

This chemical occurs naturally in some wood products, but its industrial application as rocket fuel creates sites with high ground pollution and, eventually, water pollution. Perchlorate can cause thyroid disruption in the body by substituting its chlorine atoms for the thyroid hormone's iodine. In fact, it was once used in children as a medicine to treat an overactive thyroid (hyperthyroidism). Normal thyroid hormone levels are essential for normal fetal and infant development. When perchlorate was discovered in a powdered infant formula in 2009, this serious problem was quickly remedied. I have heard little about perchlorate since that flare-up.

Phthalates

If you lisp, you can pronounce phthalates. Phthalates are widely used in many capacities and in great amounts. They are added to certain plastics, polyvinyl chloride (PCV) as in piping, to increase flexibility, and to other plastics to make them clear. They don't chemically bind with the plastic, which allows them to leach out and become water pollutants that can then enter the food chain. These chemicals have wide applications as an ingredient in products ranging from paint and pesticides to household products such as shampoos and soaps. Infants and toddlers are not going to have significant exposure to these products. What should get our attention is the fact that, unfortunately, they are hormone disrupters that act like surrogate estrogens, which can affect the normal sexual development of the fetus. Maternal exposure should therefore be considered. Obvious signs of abnormality include male infants with small penises and/or undescended testicles. One well-conducted study supports the idea of a more subtle change resulting from exposure—the altering of the brain to express more feminine characteristics. Male toddlers usually prefer to play aggressively with toys—to go "varoom" with a play truck—rather than play quietly with dolls, mimicking mother. So this characteristic can be a rather alarming signal of such exposure. Physical problems can be partially corrected with time, surgery, or medicine. Behavioral problems that may result from exposure require proper child rearing and counseling.[2]

In the November 11, 2009, issue of the *International Journal of Andrology,* Dr. Shanna Swan put forth an alarming attention-getting theory, based on her study, that young boys who had been subjected to these chemicals *in utero* showed less male typical play. This would suggest that the chemical altered "androgen responsive brain development."[3]

Perfluorinated Compounds

Problems derived from these compounds will not make the news on television. They will pop up in women's magazines as their editors search for lurking, "alarming" dangers. They have found broad application in industry because they make materials oil, water, and stain resistant, and can be found in everything from nonstick cookware and clothing to food packaging. Our infants and toddlers are not likely to have significant exposure, but they are highly persistent and have made their way into food and water and the food chain—I presume from manufacturing sites. Like phthalates, studies conducted with women show that they are hormone disrupters. A seemingly unconnected, but well-conducted study points to a diminished antibody response in children to tetanus and diphtheria vaccination. The study was conducted in an area along the Norwegian Sea, where fish contamination with these compounds is high. Children (five-year-olds) with high levels in their blood showed this depressed immune function, while children with low levels did not.[4]

The toxicity of fluoridated compounds is discussed in the fluoride chapter.

Pesticides (Including Herbicides)

The industry categorizes herbicides as included in the overall term "pesticides". An entire book could be written on the subject of the profound consequences of pesticide exposure. Hundreds of studies point to certain pesticides as having carcinogenic (cancer causing) and teratogenic (deformity producing) properties. Numerous studies point to the association of pesticide exposure and childhood cancer—leukemia, brain cancers, and non-Hodgkin's lymphoma. When cancer occurs in adults, due to a long latent period—from the first toxic insult to a few cells until the time of detectable cancer—finding *the* culprit is difficult, because there are so many possibilities that exist when one lives in a toxic environment. Cancer that appears in a toddler has bypassed that long dormant period, which makes it easier to pin down the instigator. If there could be a good side to a childhood cancer, it is this: Since it developed in a relatively short time, acute lymphocytic leukemia in a youngster is more responsive to treatment.

Ironically, childhood cancer occurs not just in the children of farm workers but in the households of highly (but poorly) educated, conscientious parents who have been led to believe that any living thing in the house that flies or scurries along the floor is harmful to children and should be *eliminated* by pesticide application. Seemingly, pesticide manufactures put conscience aside, advertise their products for household use, and put them in easy-to-use spray guns, flea collars, or lawn fertilizers that kill dandelions, and give no thought of the real possibility that there can be absorption of their chemicals through bare feet or the bare paws of the family pet.

SUMMARY

Our government agencies, which were designed to look out for our safety, seem to be foot-dragging as they recognize problems but do little about enforcing regulations. In their defense, I would suggest that there might be a reason for this: It is estimated there are "nearly 80,000 chemicals on the market. Many have not been studied, or have been understudied, and have not been regulated."[5] This same panel recommends what should be obvious—stop bad results from developing by being *precautionary* rather than *reactionary*: These agencies should do more in the line of educating the public and put less attention on enforcing regulations. As long as the public enjoys being worried, the media is going to assuage its appetite with scary half-truths. These toxic substances are cumulative—a single exposure, except in a suicide attempt, won't kill—so we need to know how they can enter our bodies and determine what are "safe" levels over time. And we need to recognize that infants and toddlers require special standards, as they are more vulnerable to these hazardous substances. What we need to learn of is the power of good nutrition and the use of vitamin supplements that mitigate the toxic action of these chemicals. Of course, as this book shows, vitamin supplements are not limited to this function alone but provide a wide variety of additional health benefits.

CHAPTER 16

DISPENSING WITH FLUORIDE

The phosphate mine that supplied our local fertilizer company was adjacent to a nearby chemical fertilizer plant that sent extracted fluoride out its chimney. This discharge polluted and poisoned adjacent fields and resulted in cattle with brittle bone disease. Witnessing this made everything I (RKC) had learned about fluoride in my public health capacity and in my private pediatric practice fit together. I have concluded that anyone who thinks fluoridating public water supplies is a good idea is simply poorly informed. There was such a public health blitz for a long time—and it was effective. Fluoridation was almost sacred. It is amazing how stubborn (or obtuse) those government bodies have been. We are opposed to fluoridation of water, a practice that is neither safe nor effective.

FLUORIDE AS "MODERN" SCIENCE

My professional life changed when I took an honest look at fluoridation of water supplies and the prescribing of fluoride to infants. There was such a push, in the 1960s, from august bodies such as the American Dental Society and my beloved American Academy of Pediatrics (AAP), to promote fluoride as the savior of children's teeth. Any physician who didn't join up was labeled as a traitor, unscientific, not fit to be a doctor, or downright un-American. The "science" of fluoride as it applies to infants and toddlers was, and is, grossly flawed. Fluoride is considered a trace mineral. Trace minerals such as magnesium, zinc, and selenium are essential for health, but only in *trace* amounts. Too much is toxic. Healthful intakes have been determined for other trace minerals, but not for fluoride.

The standard for fluoridation of public water sources, which was only very recently lowered a bit, was set at one part per million (1ppm or 1mg/liter). No attention was paid to the individual consumption of treated water. A toddler and a blast-furnace operator would drink from the same faucet water and gain vastly different intakes of fluoride. This puzzled me, because a physician should never think of prescribing a medication in liquid form and tell his patients to take whatever amount that thirst dictated.

Then, the AAP went overboard in an attempt at formulating a vitamin-fluoride drop for infants, since the breast- or bottle-fed infant would not be consuming much fluoridated water. For some time, fluoride was prescribed as part of a prenatal vitamin-mineral product. After a few years, however, some thought began to be entertained concerning a possible association between fluoride consumption and the high incidence of mottling of dental enamel that was being observed. The baby-teeth central incisors begin calcification in the fifth fetal month and is complete at eighteen to twenty-four months of age. Eruption (emergence of teeth) occurs at five to eight months. Mottling (chalky white spots) seen early can be related to maternal intake of fluoride; later on, to intake in early infancy. A stronger alarm was set off when "fluorosis" began to be more common in the permanent incisors—right in the middle of a smile.

The recommended "safe" intake was frequently adjusted. Pediatricians were admonished to calculate and adjust total fluoride intake by checking the infant's water source (still not worrying about the intake volume) and prescribing one of several different supplement drops containing different strengths of fluoride. When it was pointed out that other natural food sources of fluoride should be included in the equation, and that powdered formulas were usually reconstituted with tap water, and how much fluoride toothpaste was swallowed, the reply was, "We can't do that," backed by this statement from the AAP's 1985 edition of the *Pediatric Nutrition Handbook:* "Because these sources of fluoride are so variable, they can not be reliably estimated for any patient. Neither can water consumption, which can vary tremendously from one child to another."[1] Did they finally get it? The recommendations went on to say that calculating the proper dose should be based on body weight, but that this would be too complicated. "Therefore the dosage regimen is geared to the patient's age *for simplicity*."[2] Just when I thought the experts "got it," they threw science aside, because applying science to the problem was too complicated.

Ingestion of toothpaste was an obvious problem, but at the same time there was promotion of "fluoride swishes." Fluoride is part of the nearly impervious dental enamel. The middle-of-the-smile incisors are calcified by nine to ten years of age. The only good derived from a yearly swish would be a one-day killing effect on cariogenic bacteria in the plaque along the gumline, in children under the age of ten. A tiny amount of toothpaste teamed with proper brushing will do the same thing every day. There are other toxic effects, but the cosmetic effects get the most attention. At the same time, all this focus on fluoride has usurped the value of old fashioned dental hygiene and healthy dental nutrition: Sweep away the sticky sugary and starchy food substances that nourish cavity-forming bacteria—with or without toothpaste, or toothpaste with or without fluoride. If fluoride toothpaste is used, use only enough to "flavor" the brush. Provide tooth-building and bone-building nutrients in optimal amounts—calcium, magnesium, vitamin C, and vitamin D.

I definitely went against the grain with my letters to the AAP, our State Dental Department, and to local newspapers. I had previously supplied the city administrators of a nearby town, who desired to remain without fluoridation, with information about its drawbacks. At the decision-making hearing, I was met not only by the State Dental Officer but, sadly, several of my pediatric colleagues who were determined to "set me straight." Ironically, I was a respected member of the Board of our State Chapter of the AAP at the time. I soon learned of "ignorance in high places" in regards to gaining and applying nutrition knowledge.

The significance of dental fluorosis is that it is the canary in the mine. It becomes a legal issue because this litigious culture accommodates fixing blame wherever it can. Parents spend thousands on orthodonture work to give their children perfect teeth only to find chalky white spots on the teeth in the middle of their smile. Little attention is given to other effects of fluorosis, such as the brittle bone disease in the cattle near the belching chimney of a chemical phosphate fertilizer plant, or the story of dumping fluoride—the waste product of fertilizer production—into public water supplies.

FLUORIDE AS A "BELIEF SYSTEM"

I found that the one and only still actively practicing pediatrician in our "big" city had not a clue about the value or harm from prescribed infant vitamins that contained fluoride. He just blindly followed the AAP recommendation. In our book *The Vitamin Cure for Children's Health Problems,* we discuss all the dosage gyrations the AAP went through in order to keep prescribing fluoride for infants in an amount that would not produce fluorosis, caused by overexposure to fluoride, most apparent as dental fluorosis. Parents need to educate themselves so they can be prepared with a suitable argument when they refuse fluoride-containing vitamin preparations. Mothers, for sure, are going to be confronted with this pressure from their pediatricians. If refusal might cause pediatric excommunication, we recommend this: Accept the prescription, don't fill it, do your homework, *then* decide whether to fill it or not.

As a child, there was nothing I (AWS) liked about going to the dental dispensary, with the possible exception of the large tropical fish aquarium in the waiting room. This was a distraction from what was coming: three hours in a vast hall containing a double line of black dental chairs and a matching double line of white-clad dental students. And that, as a six-year-old, is where I first encountered fluoride on a regular basis. After a free cleaning and checkup (the reason my cost-conscious parents had me go to the dispensary, and the reason it literally took three hours to complete), fluoride was applied to my teeth with a swab. I remember both the smell (acrid) and the taste (astringent). I actually looked forward to the fluoride treatment, simply because it was the last thing they did to me before I was allowed to leave. Did it work? Probably not. In addition to my regular topical fluoride treatments, I lived in a city with fluoridated water and was raised on fluoridated toothpaste. And I had a mouthful of amalgam by my high-school graduation.

Controversy? What Controversy?

In the late 1970s, as a young parent, I (AWS) became aware of the *National Fluoridation News,* published in the still largely unknown town of Gravette, Arkansas (pop 2,200). For a very small donation, I received a boxful of back issues by return mail. In addition to this generosity, what surprised me about the *NFNews* was the high caliber of its content. Most of the noneditorial articles were well referenced and the work of well qualified scientists. This was something of a poser, for as a college biology major, I had been thoroughly schooled in the two Noble Truths of Fluoridation: (1) that fluoride in drinking water would reduce tooth decay by 60 to 65 percent; and (2) that anyone who disagreed with this view was a fool. Yes, I had seen the movie *Dr. Strangelove,* and yes, I knew how to read an American Dental Association (ADA) endorsement on a toothpaste label.

Not long after this, my penchant for reading toothpaste labels paid off. There it was, printed right on the back of the tube:

> Children should only use a "pea-sized" portion of fluoride toothpaste when they brush.

I had two toddlers, and this caught my interest. Looking into it, I learned that small children swallow a considerable quantity of toothpaste when they brush, perhaps most of it.

Anyone who has watched television at all could not have failed to see toothpaste ads. They always showed the brush loaded with toothpaste, embellished with decorative overhang tips flared out on each end. When Aim brand toothpaste first came out, I distinctly remember toothpaste being displayed in two or even three layers on the brush. The number of children that used the product so generously, and swallowed half of it, will likely remain unknown. As for me, I immediately switched my family to toothpaste with no fluoride in it. As for toothpaste labels, they rather quickly were rewritten. They now read:

If you accidentally swallow more than used for brushing, seek
professional help or contact a poison control center immediately.

But *all* children swallow more than is used for brushing. The only
question is, how much? The US Centers for Disease Control states:

> Fluoride toothpaste contributes to the risk for enamel fluoro-
> sis because the swallowing reflex of children aged less than
> 6 years is not always well controlled, particularly among
> children aged less than 3 years. Children are also known to
> swallow toothpaste deliberately when they like its taste. A
> child-sized toothbrush covered with a full strip of toothpaste
> holds approximately 0.75–1.0 g of toothpaste, and each gram
> of fluoride toothpaste, as formulated in the United States, con-
> tains approximately 1.0 mg of fluoride. *Children aged less than
> 6 years swallow a mean of 0.3 g of toothpaste per brushing and
> can inadvertently swallow as much as 0.8 g.*[3] (emphasis added)

For children age six and under, that is an *average* swallow of a third
of the toothpaste they use, and a possibility of inadvertently swallowing 80 percent or more. There is about a milligram of fluoride in a single "serving" of toothpaste. I am calling it a "serving" because fluoride
in toothpaste is regulated as if it were a food, not a drug. How is this
true? Adding even less than one milligram of fluoride to a single serving of children's vitamins instantly makes them a prescription drug. It is
truly odd that fluoride toothpaste remains an over-the-counter product.

Dr. Campbell adds: Few toddlers have mastered the fine art of collecting the contents of the mouth, then spitting it out—especially if the
contents taste good. The exception might be the infant or toddler who
enjoys "food fights." Both spitting and nose blowing require a certain
maturity of the nervous system.

Into the Schools

When my (AWS) children were in grade school, the local dental college
(the people who brought us the dispensary I went to as a young boy)
interested our school district in a research project. Our town's public
water was under local control and unfluoridated, unlike the city

nearby. So the idea was to administer fluoride rinses to schoolchildren, during the school day, and then count caries. We were asked to sign a permission letter, which emphasized likely benefits and glossed over any hazards. Remembering what youngsters did with sweet toothpaste, I made a guess that they'd swallow a saccharin-laced rinse about as well. We chose to not sign. But I did check the box to receive results of the study. It ultimately came in the form of a letter, saying that the results were disappointingly inconclusive: no evidence that fluoride rinses helped our unfluoridated-water-drinking community. I am unaware whether the study was published.

That is not especially surprising. Shutting out access to balanced scientific discussion of fluoridation is alive and well . . . and taxpayer supported. Negative fluoride studies and reviews are hardly abundant on PubMed/MEDLINE. One does not need to be a conspiracy theorist to observe that the U.S. National Library of Medicine refuses to index the journal *Fluoride*.[4] (Censorship is conspicuously aberrant behavior for any public library. If you want access to what the U.S. taxpayer-funded National Library of Medicine refuses to index, you may read over forty years' of articles from the journal *Fluoride*, free of charge, at http://www.fluorideresearch.org/. Scroll down to "Archives and Indexes, 1968–2011.") Albert W. Burgstahler, Ph.D. comments: "Support for these views and conclusions is found in a recent review in *Critical Public Health* titled 'Slaying Sacred Cows: Is It Time to Pull the Plug on Water Fluoridation?'[5] by Stephen Peckham of the Department of Health Services Research and Policy, London School of Hygiene and Tropical Medicine. In his article, Peckham concludes that evidence for the effectiveness and safety of water fluoridation is seriously defective and not in agreement with findings of a growing body of current and previously overlooked research."

No Discussion

About fifteen years ago, our (AWS) town's public water supply was annexed by the nearby metropolis. Aside from a rate increase, the only other, barely detectable change to our bill was a one-time typed legend at the bottom stating that fluoride has now been added to the water.

There had been no vote, and there had not even been any discussion. Communities coast-to-coast know that this is not at all uncommon.

Four glasses of fluoridated tap water contain about as much fluoride as a prescription dose does. Not only is fluoridated water nonprescription, it is even more certain to be swallowed than toothpaste. Being over six years of age means better control over swallowing reflexes, thus limiting ingestion of fluoride from toothpaste. There is no such accommodation for drinking water.

Evidence-based medicine requires evidence before medicating. Fluoridation of water is not evidence-based. It has not been tested in well-controlled studies. Fluoridation of public water is a default medication, since you have to deliberately avoid it if you do not want to take it. A person's daily intake of fluoride simply from drinking an average quantity of fluoridated tap water, fluoridated bottled water, and beverages produced or prepared with fluoridated water can easily exceed the threshold that your druggist would rightly demand for a prescription. Fluoride in toothpaste and mouth rinses is also medication. It may be intended as topical, but the reality is different. No matter how it is applied in their mouths, young children are going to swallow it. Indeed, most of the public and the dental profession already have.

To Fluoridate or Not to Fluoridate

The whole fluoridation issue has been a big part of my (RKC) separate stance from conventional medicine—not to be ornery, but in an attempt to counter all the untruths out there about it. My father fought fluoridation tooth and nail (in the late 1950s and 1960s, no less). I got lots of flack related to my views on fluoride-rinse swishing from a state dental officer.

Since dental enamel is incapable of absorbing *any* substance, how could topical fluoride have anything to do with cavity prevention or tooth formation? I did find that topical fluoride inhibited bacterial growth at the gum-line. For this activity toothpaste is as effective as swishing, and is utilized more often. Proper tooth brushing with a vertical rather than horizontal sweeping action would probably fill the bill. Getting cariogenic foods (cavity-promoting foods such as gooey sugary things, even dried fruit) off the teeth soon after contact is helpful.

"Medicating water" brings up a basic issue. How did the authorities arrive at the precise concentration of fluoride in drinking water? Intake of this "active ingredient" would vary infinitely with body weight or activity. Would a blast-furnace worker and a baby be having a similar intake of fluoride?

Oddly enough, my agricultural experience revealed the origins of fluoridation. Using fluoride is a way to get rid of this toxic stuff that was derived from the making of phosphate fertilizers. The sad thing was the prescribing of fluoride drops, prenatally and for infants. It took decades for change to come about. By recognizing the mottling of enamel as a sign of toxicity, public outcry got some improvements in prescribing fluoride drops and, finally, in reducing the concentration in public water supplies. There has been harmful foot-dragging by the authoritative bodies. In spite of my being on the Board of the Montana Chapter of the AAP, my colleagues and the state dentist showed up with fire in their eyes at a meeting when I spoke against fluoridation of the St. Ignatius water supply. I was a "Commie" from then on. Their ignorance was palpable. I endured, even prevailed, but I was permanently out of the old boy's network, with great loss of credibility.

REVERSING FLUOROSIS

Although visible tooth mottling is likely irreversible, vitamin C seems to greatly assist the liver in recovering from excess fluoride intake.

"Amongst the various antidotes, ascorbic acid (vitamin C) was the most beneficial in bringing about pronounced recovery, followed vitamin E and calcium. However, all three antidotes administered together resulted in significant recovery in the histoarchitecture (tissue structure) and carbohydrate metabolism of liver and serum transaminases."[1]

Reference

1. Nair, S. B., D. D. Jhala, N. J. Chinoy. "Beneficial Effects of Certain Antidotes in Mitigating Fluoride and/or Arsenic Induced Hepatotoxicity in Mice." *Fluoride* 35(4) (2002):60–70. http://www.fluorideresearch.org/372/files/FJ2004_v37_n2_p60–70.pdf (accessed Nov 2012).

Is it all over now? Ralph Nader has come out against water fluoridation. The U.S. Centers for Disease Control and Prevention admit that 41 percent of twelve- to fifteen-year-olds, and 36 percent of sixteen- to nineteen-year-olds have dental fluorosis (tooth mottling). In January 2011, the U.S. Department of Health and Human Services recommended a reduction of fluoride in drinking water. Has fluoridation finally been foiled?

If so, it's been a long process. Back in 1980, when my children were infants, I (AWS) noticed that virtually every country in Europe had stopped fluoridation. A few years later, I read an article in *Chemical and Engineering News* that a review of the research showed that people who have grown up with fluoridated water have, on average, only one-half of one filling less per lifetime than people who did not drink fluoridated water.[7]

So I am biased, having set my proverbial teeth against fluoridation long ago. My children were raised in a community without water fluoridation, without fluoride mouth rinses, and using fluoride-free toothpaste. My son had a cavity and my daughter had three cavities . . . total, through all their teen years. That is not proof, but it is certainly a little intriguing. (It is also evidence of the nutritional aspects of good health, since dental health, like general health, can not be attributed to just one nutrient.)

But talk about intrigue: The real story started in the 1940s and fluoridation trials began in 1945. The U.S. Public Health Service endorsed fluoridation on June 1, 1950 . . . before any trials were completed. Endorsements from the American Dental Association and the American Public Health Association followed before year's end. This "ready, fire, aim" approach was the mother of the claim, which I repeatedly heard as a child and as a parent, that water fluoridation would reduce dental caries by 90 percent. I have seen no evidence to support this claim, or even that it reduced cavities by a reasonable fraction of that figure. Indeed, some regions of the United States with nearly universal water fluoridation have the most decayed, missing, and filled teeth in the nation.

The whole sordid affair is detailed, with energy and rigorous scholarship, in an excellent book, *The Case Against Fluoride*. The authors offer considerably more than many readers ever wanted to know about the subject. That is a compliment. This is certainly information all should know, and almost certainly did not. Sections in the book include a history of fluoridation, evidence of ineffectiveness, evidence of harm, safety issues, ethical arguments, and, perhaps most scathing, an inside look at fluoridation promotion techniques. It is a partisan presentation. It is also heavily, even relentlessly, substantiated, with eighty pages of references. Ignoring such an array of literature is the only way to dismiss it.

The orthomolecular community is divided on this issue. Water fluoridation might be considered orthomolecular, the practice being a medical use of a substance normally found in the human body. Linus Pauling is said to have supported water fluoridation. On the other hand, fluoridation might be considered toximolecular, since even moderate overconsumption of fluoride not only causes dental fluorosis but has also been shown to be associated with an increase incidence of osteosarcoma and other diseases.[7,8] Significantly, "too much" is a small increase, sometimes a matter of only a fraction of a milligram per liter in excess of water concentrations generally recognized as safe. All fluoride supplements, including fluoridated vitamins, should require a prescription. I am puzzled by this. Even those in orthomolecular medicine should admit that their original stance has proven to be *wrong*.

In 1990, Abram Hoffer commented on John Yiamouyiannis' analysis[9] of US Public Health Service data. "(F)luoridation had no significant

FLUORIDE AND IQ

In August 2012, Philippe Grandjean, M.D., Ph.D., from the Department of Environmental Health, Harvard School of Public Health, published about a research project conducted jointly with China Medicine University on the association of fluoride concentrations and IQ. China has natural fluoridation, with a wide variation of concentrations from one area to the other. "Children living in highly fluoridated areas had significantly lower IQ scores than their peers living in areas of low fluoridation." Dr. Grandjean further commented that, "Fluoride seems to fit in with lead, mercury, and other poisons that cause brain drain."

effect on children's teeth," Dr. Hoffer wrote, adding that "studies showing fluoride is carcinogenic (capable of inducing cancer) and non-therapeutic when added to water provides support to the 'unscientific' views of fluoride opponents."[10]

Fluoridation is alive and presumed well in the majority of America's faucets. Is the fluoridation debate over? Those in favor of fluoridation typically say yes, and for some time now. The authors disagree. Declaring a victory by ignoring research is politics, not science.

There is not a great deal of published academic debate on the topic. Yiamouyiannis' paper, mentioned above, appeared in the journal *Fluoride*. MEDLINE steadfastly refuses to index *Fluoride*, even though it is peer reviewed, balanced in coverage of the topic, and has been continuously published for forty-four years. Many readers will not find this all that surprising. The entire *Fluoride* archive is online for free access at http://www.fluorideresearch.org/.

"Balance" is a word that has never been welcome in the fluoride debate. Citizens and scientists critical of fluoridation have been and still are dismissed as cranks. It is curious that so many anti-antifluoride articles cite the movie *Dr. Strangelove* to bolster their arguments for fluoridation. The movie was a work of fiction. *The Case Against Fluoride* offers much evidence that to assert that fluoridation of water is safe and effective is a fiction as well.

REVERSING THE FLUORIDATION TREND

There recently been successful rescinding of fluoridation in several major American cities whose water supplies were formerly fluoridated. It takes a lot of effort to get city commissioners to look at the facts and take this bold action. Portland, Oregon, at the time of this writing, is currently going through this process. I contacted my niece, Lynne Campbell, knowing that she, while working with Dr. Lendon Smith, had an active part in thwarting the initial push to fluoridate Portland. She told me about the money behind the push for fluoridation, and how the backers attempt to flood the final decision makers with questionable studies. She also told me of some of the more obscure sources of fluoride and their significance, such as grapes. I knew that grapes received increased amounts of pesticides, which I assumed would be fungicides (technically, fungicides, herbicides, and insecticides are all called pesticides) because of mildew affecting the broad leaves. She described the different toxicity of the different forms of fluoride. Sodium fluoride was the original type used in fluoridation, but currently the more chemically active silicofluorides are used 90 percent of the time. Children in fluoridated areas have two times the blood lead levels of those in areas without fluoridation.

She thought that Andrew Young's statement (below) was interesting, and that because of his stature as former United Nations Ambassador and former Atlanta Mayor, he might be heard. Ambassador Young felt that our government would rather just back public water fluoridation instead of supporting useful health programs for poor black kids that would improve their nutritional status. In his letter to the Georgia Legislature he addresses the fact that current science shows fluoride's primary effect to be topical, not systemic.

> . . . My father was a dentist. I formerly was a strong believer in the benefits of water fluoridation for preventing cavities. But many things that we began to do 50 or more years ago we now no longer do, because we have learned further information that changes our practices and policies. So it is with fluoridation. We originally thought people needed to swallow it, so the fluoride would be incorporated into teeth before they erupted from the gums. Our belief in the need for systemic absorption was why we began adding fluoride to drinking water. But now we know that the primary, limited cavity fighting effects of fluoride are topical, when fluorides touch teeth in the mouth. We know that fluorides do little to stop cavities where they occur most often, in the pits and fissures of the back molars where food packs down into the grooves. This is why there is a big push today to use teeth sealants in the molars of children. We also have a cavity epidemic today in our inner cities that have been fluoridated for decades. . . ."
>
> —Andrew Young, Letter to Chip Rogers, Senate Majority Leader, Georgia State Capital, March 29, 2011

The Fluoride Action Network

In my effort to find references to Lynne's information, I found a very worthwhile website while searching under "fluoride sources." This marvelous resource is the Fluoride Action Network (www.fluoridealert.org). To quote from their site: "The problem with fluoride, therefore, is not that children are receiving too little, but that they are receiving too much." Reducing the fluoride safety levels of water will do nothing when put against the inadvertent intake from our environment. The Fluoride Action Network shows a graph of the incidence of dental fluorosis in fifteen-year-olds, which is striking and pathetic: 23 percent from 1986–1987, rising to 41 percent from 1999–2004. They also explain the grape (and other vegetable, fruit, fruit drink, and wine) source of fluoride, which proved to be cryolite (sodium hexafluoroaluminate) used as an insecticide, resulting in over twice the level of fluoride found in fluoridated water. (This can be avoided by using organic products.) We have mentioned the intake from mixing baby powdered milk formula with fluoridated water, but there is a more subtle problem in many processed foods and beverages. Drying fruits greatly concentrates any pesticide residue. Another interesting report available on the site describes a study by Professor Roger D. Masters at Dartmouth College. It is unique in that it can explain (in my opinion) the association of lead levels, influenced by fluorides, and ADHD and lowered IQ. His thesis suggests that violent behavior can have its origin in elevated blood-lead levels that depress dopa formation (the precursor to other neurotransmitters) by the silicofluoride's ability to increase absorption of lead from the environment.

NOTE TO READERS

Some material in this chapter first appeared in the journal *Fluoride*, published by the International Society for Fluoride Research, http://www.fluorideresearch.org. It is reprinted with permission.

For Further Reading

Connett, P., J. Beck, H. Spedding Micklem. *The Case Against Fluoride: How Hazardous Waste Ended Up in Our Drinking Water and the Bad Science and Powerful Politics That Keep It There.* VT: Chelsea Green Publishing, 2010.

CHAPTER 17

PEDIATRICIANS AND PEDIATRICS

Parents are going to wonder, "Where are the orthomolecular pediatricians? Is there one near me?" The answer is, probably not. The only way you will know for sure is to ask friends, ask at local health food stores, and especially, search the Internet. There must be some out there somewhere. There are advantages to having a physician who can juggle the restraints of our insurance system and still provide an orthomolecular concept of good care. We hope you can find a few and question them. We hate the idea that nutritional medicine might be available only for the rich. In my (RKC) area it was impossible for me to be an effective orthomolecular doctor or to call myself one. I went to marvelous educational conferences, such as Orthomolecular Medicine Today, when I could. I applied what I learned in those meetings and also from several Environmental Medicine meetings, to my private practice and to my public health duties. I was happy to do it, but it is tough to make a living when there is no charge, since health care insurance, of course, would not reimburse me.

A specialist physician could embrace our ideas and apply them in his or her advice to patients, or even provide intravenous vitamin C to patients since the overall fee is assured by having had the necessary referral from a primary care physician. As we pointed out in our book *The Vitamin Cure for Children's Health* the primary care physician makes a living only by following guidelines of care set out by the insurance company that covers his or her practice. Unlike Jesus' admonition, "Be in the world but not of it," it is hard not to be "of it" in this medical world. Most doctors are so certain of what is "proper" care that they are super-sensitive about a parent telling them (or even suggesting) what to do. I know that if, in this book, I told a mother to tell her doctor to check out megadoses of vitamin C, it would cause swift and thorough excommunication for her. For this very reason, I hope this book will be something of a primer for open-minded physicians, to help them provide reasonable answers for their patient's questions.

I am especially intrigued by Dr. Robert Cathcart's and Dr. Hugh Riordan's use of intravenous (IV) vitamin C. (see Chapter 14). I knew about it in the past, and I knew that it worked because of the source of the information. It seems to me that Dr. Cathcart had a philosophy like Dr. Lendon Smith's when he stated that he treated some things with an appropriate antibiotic *plus* vitamin C at bowel tolerance levels. I did use the "bowel tolerance" concept but, in the restricted environment of my practice, had no way of administering IV vitamin C myself. Nor did I know any of my physician contacts who would be able to use this information. In my training, I figured out many ways to get IV fluids into an infant through all kinds of tiny veins, but it isn't easy.

Here is where oral dosing of vitamin C comes in mighty handy: parents can and have done it, as the Chapter 14 explains. I have tried to provide common sense approaches to many of the problems of infants. They worked then and they work now.

The authors thoroughly agree on a three-tier approach for children: (1) A good diet and a multivitamin, at a minimum; (2) special vitamin supplements for special needs; and (3) high orthomolecular doses when appropriate. What we have attempted to do is to write on what we have learned: from the literature and what we have seen from our different professional backgrounds. We write about things we have had hands-on experience with—the only things we have proven to our satisfaction—that work.

REFLECTIONS OF AN OLD CODGER

I had enjoyed my special privileges of *emeritus* status in the American Academy of Pediatrics (AAP), which included reduced fees to meetings and a free subscription to the journal *Pediatrics* when suddenly I was told that there would be no more free subscription and that I needed to pay my dues immediately. I was no longer in active practice but I wanted to continue playing an active part in pediatric education, so I wrote a letter with the tongue-in-cheek title "Reflections of an Old Codger" you see above—though I hoped the contents would not be taken lightly. I stipulated that if my letter would be presented to the higher authorities and I received a response from them, I would pay for ongoing membership. If not, what was the need for continuing? I had presented letters in the past on the subjects presented in the letter. Some were published or I got a response back; not so with others. My swan song was not answered. Thus endeth my membership.

I began a correspondence with Ms. Sally Bunday in June of 1994. She was an executive for an organization in England, HACSG (the hyperactive children's support group for hyperactive, allergic and learning-disabled children—thank goodness for acronyms). I was referred to her by Dr. William Crook, who suggested that I could best give the "U.S." view—knowing full well that he and I were in solid agreement concerning the etiology of these issues. I was surprised to learn that her organization had been battling wrong concepts and the push for medications for seventeen years. Much of our correspondence is also included in this chapter.

I (RKC) am still wrestling with the concept of a children's doctor of today. Now aged eighty-five, I have always been one who goes against the grain, but, as I reflect, the atmosphere has changed. I enjoyed my colleagues and they enjoyed me. Sometimes I would come around to their way of thinking, and sometimes they would come around to mine. One never considered the other as a screw ball.

I simply suggest not forgetting to look at the past, to avoid discarding what worked. My realization of the complete schism between my concept of pediatrics and the current one expressed in *Pediatrics* (and the media's interpretations of its articles) has led me to consider surrendering my membership in the American Association of Pediatrics—an organization I have been so proud of.

The fun of solving and getting at the basis of pediatric problems has been taken away by constraints on the amount of time doctors can spend with patients, and a shift of faith from clinical observation and experience to tests and pharmaceuticals. We tell children to "just say no to drugs," yet encourage their use for every ill, real or imagined. We might as well adopt the commercial slogan, "Just do it!" Committees, consisting of experts, set the standards of care. They tell us how we are to counsel and prescribe for children as they face choices of lifestyle, covering issues such as sexual orientation and substance abuse or objectionable behavior. "Choice" has become the keyword, supplanting any idea of right or wrong that might be imparted by an individual practitioner.

The Rise of Prescriptions and Imprecise Diagnoses

The distinction between drugs and medicines has always been blurred, depending more on whether a substance is prescribed or illicit. We used to go to the drug store for our medicines. We have a drug or medicine for everything, tried and proven tangible diagnoses, as well as ambiguous "behavioral disorders." For a psychotropic drug to sell, physicians have to be convinced of its value first, then parents (or "caretakers"), but the recipient children have no say in their treatment. True underlying causes of disturbing behavior cannot be sought within the time constraints of a brief office visit evaluation, nor can any meaningful rapport be established that allows for a trusting doctor-patient interaction. A conjured-up diagnosis best fitting the undesirable behavior that parents and their physician (within the allotted time slot) have observed, perhaps augmented by observations or anecdotal reports from teachers or the school nurse, has to satisfy. The next step is to get the precise drug for this imprecise diagnosis.

Allow me to illustrate what I mean by imprecise diagnosis. The history of attention deficit disorder (ADD) or attention deficit hyperactivity disorder (ADHD) is revealing. Around the late 1950s a number of simultaneous changes started happening in our society: an expanded presence of television; mothers finding distractions from child rearing, such as jobs and interests outside of the home; and the introduction of massive amounts of sugar and processed foods into our children's diets. About that same time, pediatricians and school personnel began to be concerned that many children, some of whom wiggled a lot, could or would not pay attention. The subtle changes occurring in our culture were not recognized as factors that could detract from the *learned* process of acquiring attention span. The preschooler no longer matriculated from sitting still on mother's lap while looking at picture books to reading along with her. And many emerging experts dismissed what teachers observed as "mad November first" after a night of trick or treating and sugar ingestion.

NUTRITIONAL SUPPLEMENTS REDUCE ANTISOCIAL BEHAVIOR

"Experimental, double-blind, placebo-controlled, randomised trial of nutritional supplements on 231 young adult prisoners, comparing disciplinary offences before and during supplementation. Compared with placebos, those receiving the active capsules committed an average of 26.3 percent (95 percent CI 8.3–44.33 percent) fewer offences. Compared to baseline, the effect on those taking active supplements for a minimum of two weeks. Antisocial behaviour in prisons, including violence, are reduced by vitamins, minerals, and essential fatty acids with similar implications for those eating poor diets in the community."[1]

Reference

1. Gesch, C. B., S. M. Hammond, S. E. Hampson, et al. "Influence of Supplementary Vitamins, Minerals and Essential Fatty Acids on the Antisocial Behaviour of Young Adult Prisoners. Randomised, Placebo-Controlled Trial." *Br J Psychiatry.* 181 (2002):22–28.

Since it was un-American to blame mothers or the marvels of science as applied to developing new "easy" foods, and we were not yet able to comprehend the drawbacks of television, we invented a medical problem that required a medical solution, and thereby circumvented a search for real causes and more cumbersome solutions. It was first called "minimal brain dysfunction." I believe that I was in on the genesis of the behavioral syndromes in the late 1950s, being in a Southern California college town. Within a short span of time, I witnessed many name changes: "hyperkinetic child syndrome," "minimal brain damage," "minimal cerebral dysfunction," (note the upgrade from "brain" to "cerebral"—a real scientific ring to it). Motivation for a continuing search for the proper term seemed to be driven by the desire to convince the public that the diagnosis was as rock-solid as "lobar pneumonia." Collaborative tests of motor function, looking for so-called "soft neurological signs" that would support the diagnosis, were in vogue: patient pointer finger to examiner's pointer finger; patient's pointer finger to patient's nose; and patient's hands slapping patient's thighs, alternating between the dorsal and ventral aspects of the hands, in rapid succession (one of my favorites). Of course any patient could perform these tests well if given enough time. To be significantly abnormal, the physician had to have some objective standard of speed of operation in mind. The physician's speed was the usual benchmark. Some of us asked, "So what do we do with these deviations from what is supposedly normal?" The answer, apparently, was to *treat*. Providing a stressed parent with a tangible diagnosis and a tangible treatment avoided a lot of introspection and feelings of inadequacy.

This was the beginning of the search for a drug treatment that would best fit the perceived problem. Sleepy kids can't pay attention. *These kids can't pay attention. Therefore, wake them up with a stimulant. With today's problems with amphetamine use, it would be unthinkable to kick off a treatment campaign with this powerful stimulant,* but in the early ADD days this was the first-line, and the only treatment, for narcolepsy. Very quickly a public relations campaign got underway to tout the therapeutic value of the milder stimulant, Ritalin (I use the trade name because the public never heard the generic name).

Support for this shaky syndrome came from successful public and professional involvement in the form of "educational" seminars sponsored by the pharmaceutical company that produced Ritalin. Speakers consisted of pediatric neurologists, child psychiatrists and psychologists, educators (teachers and administrators), and of course, parents who willingly gave their "testimony." Many school psychologists and teachers soon became medical experts. I had personal experience with some of these untrained people, who attributed the cause of unacceptable behavior to brain damage from obstetrical mishaps or to experiencing a high fever in infancy, and flat-out telling parents as much. Off-the-cuff diagnoses became the norm. Following the seminars primary doctors, with input from school personnel and parents, wrote prescriptions for Ritalin at an alarming rate in spite of the hollow admonitions found in the *Physicians' Desk Reference* (PDR) of not jumping in to medication treatment before conducting a thorough work-up that included input from school personnel and parents.

In the age of enlightenment that followed, in which we learned much about neurotransmitters, we still don't have a clue of how stimulants or other psychotropic drugs work in these vague syndromes. A misinformed public is apparently placated by the term "correcting a chemical imbalance," because many advertisements use this catch phrase. The PDR states that the mode of action of Ritalin and other stimulants is unknown, but that it *presumably* activates the brain stem arousal system and cortex. I have read of Ritalin's incompatibility with monoamine oxidase (MAO) inhibitors. Since MAO is involved in the catabolism of both serotonin and norepinephrine, I presume that, apart from the stimulant effect, this drug might have some effect on attention through these neurotransmitters.

Earlier in my career, the public's perception of a pediatrician attributed to him or her the know-how to provide helpful counsel for behavioral problems. High sounding diagnostic labels were shunned in favor of straight talk. The well-child check was given enough time to include what might now be called "confounding factors" that influence behavior—nutrition, exposure to environmental toxins, including food allergens, social or psychiatric problems within the family, and, of course, any intellectual or sensory deficits that a physical examination could reveal. Mutually worked out programs for resolving problems were undertaken by pediatrician and parent, and follow-up visits were scheduled. The children were included in the discussion of a treatment plan if they were old enough to understand.

I am seeing that this ideal is probably a thing of the past and cannot be resurrected, simply because medical insurance money goes for tests and pharmaceuticals and not for physician time or counsel. Other psychotropic drugs are being developed and used for equally shaky diagnoses.

Intelligent, resourceful toddlers playing "king of the mountain" with their parents, attempting manipulation and control over the bigger beings around them, are a given; but this behavior should certainly not last into the school years. We big people live in a world that *we* control. No amount of arguing or shows of defiance will change that, and the child needs to learn to get over it. If parents don't have the skill to gain back control by the time the child is ready for school, there is a problem for everyone, including the school. The common solution for those children who don't come around in time—a behavioral disorder diagnosis and a matching drug.

Something out of the *Diagnostic and Statistical Manual of Mental Health Disorders (DSM-IV)*—like "oppositional defiant disorder," matched with a prescription for a supposedly tailor-made medicine that will block an enzyme involved in neurotransmitter balance will probably not provide long-term customer satisfaction. The diagnostic label might placate the parent who is taken off the hook for lacking parenting skills, and the doctor who can now have a code for billing purposes, but to an unenlightened teacher of the "old school," the kid is still a brat and is disturbing the non-brats. Saying that ADHD may coexist with equally nebulous diagnoses in the "disruptive behavior disorders" group that can be found in the manual does not add strength to its legitimacy. A look at the description for Risperidone in the PDR, a drug recommended for the treatment of these disorders, has only a little over two columns of description and mechanism of action (and the usual for the mechanism of psychotropic drugs—*unknown,* but it is proposed that it is an antagonist to both dopamine and serotonin). The remaining ten columns are devoted to describing warnings, contraindications, and studies describing undesirable side effects. At the very least, such a drug should be relegated to the "last resort" category, especially when contemplating prescribing for a child with no ability to protest.

As long as pharmaceutical companies profit from making and promoting "quick fix" drugs and are as successful as they have been in the past in convincing the public that this is the way to go, and as long as pediatricians support this mode of action and the AAP capitulates, there will be no return to honestly addressing important life issues. I was particularly despondent after seeing an advertisement on television for a website for the Academy to answer questions about ADD and ADHD. This can hardly be interpreted as anything other than an attempt to bolster their stubborn stance of drug treatment for behavior disorders and stultify any consideration of alternative treatment or causes.

> As to "medicines," particularly over-the-counter (OTC) junk, I used to use very little of this stuff for infants. Now, I categorically say, *just say no to drugs.*

Clinical observations of what works, made by those in the trenches, should receive more attention instead of stubbornly holding to theories. The Safe to Sleep (originally Back to Sleep) program is touted for causing a dramatic decline in sudden infant death syndrome (SIDS) deaths, and a recent Cook County Hospital study leaves no stone unturned to prove that the decline is solely attributed to keeping infants on their backs (except when under scrutiny if on their tummies). Could some of the decline be due to prior emergency-room-only patients now getting well-child checks? Or their parents receiving a bit more health care advice than simply "place your infant on his/her back"—advice like, "think about the bedding, don't prevent the escape of body heat, kick smokers out of the house, call for instruction if your baby has difficulty breathing due to obstruction in any part of the airway (even just a stuffy nose)"? Is an autopsy performed to establish this diagnosis, by exclusion, for every infant death? Are we any closer than we were thirty-five years ago to finding a real cause? An expert on national TV news, recently, said that one theory was that these infants became over-heated and that is why putting them on their backs helps. That puzzled me, because many pediatricians have had great success in lowering high fevers of infants, with cool sponging of the back, with its uncontoured, expansive skin surface. I am seeing, as a nonpracticing observer, grossly (in my view) flattened infant occiputs (the back of the head) coming from this program. For that very reason, during my first year of practice with patients both in the Mexican barrio and the homes of college professors, I encouraged placing healthy babies prone on safe bedding. Out of thousands of infants in a thirteen-year period in Southern California, I had only one SIDS death, which was perhaps tobacco smoke related. There have to be other etiologic factors that make more sense. Confounding factors associated with either supine or prone positions may be the real culprit. The search should continue.

The Resistance to Open-Mindedness

Unyielding positions on such things as immunization safety and lead toxicity, as well as positions that really belong in the social sciences are very frustrating. If there continues to be an all-out effort to preserve the status quo, not just pediatrics but all of clinical medicine will die. The crisis of pediatric type 2 diabetes and childhood obesity would never have occurred if the emphasis on the importance of comprehensive well-child checks had prevailed. Nutritional advice and the encouragement of exercise can not be provided in a fifteen minute acute care visit that covers these things only in handouts. Medicines will never replace sound nutritional advice. As we speak, politicians

WATER ON THE FARM

We have, for our water source, a deep well that produces pure, cold (in the 40 degree range) drinking water—one of the reasons for our move from the end of the line for the Colorado River. On hot days of cherry harvest, I see to it that our pickers get plenty of it. This year, I found all these bottles, some full of water, a few empty, lying in the grass. Some group got a government grant to buy bottled water (from a faucet elsewhere or a contaminated, *natural* source?) and dole it out to our pickers when they get some other freebies. Yesterday, my dog came home with a bottle he had found in the orchard. It had a "Nutrition Facts" label. I was surprised to learn that water had zero total fat, zero trans fats, zero sodium, zero total carbohydrates, and zero protein. Your government watchdogs in action!

are scurrying to promise that older folks will get their umpteen drugs at a lower price than they now pay. If these patients could cut the *number* of drugs they take by 50 percent that, truly, would be a savings. Do we want to indoctrinate our pediatric patients into the same false philosophy of health care? I think not, because the financial pressures derived from "a drug for everything" is going to collapse the system of health care as we know it. Worried parents with an acutely ill child, in a rushed office environment, are not prepared to discuss the deeper issues of nutritional deficiencies, excesses, or the value of exercise and right choices.

There appears to be an almost defiant defense of immunizations. We don't have to be reminded of the unquestionable overall benefit, but there needs to be more honesty about the drawbacks, or the public will lose faith and not accept new programs. Some of us remember some of the miscues of the manufacturers and the pushes for universal immunization programs. The measles vaccination in one arm at the same time as gamma globulin in the other made no sense. We took no pleasure in saying, "I told you so" when severe measles pneumonia cases ensued. And why was the first H. *influenzae* (Hib) vaccine given, when it didn't hit the desired target age group? An early rubella vaccine caused monoarticular rheumatoid arthritis. There have been known bad batches of vaccines. The shrill, hysterical cry that persists, unabated, for hours in an infant DPT recipient—an obvious sign of neurological insult—scares the dickens out of parents and physicians alike. Yet, it is almost trivialized, as is the shocklike signs that can occur within minutes after administration. We are bombarded with articles that attempt to disprove any harm in giving multiple vaccines at one time in young infants. Never before have we had such multiples; so we can not yet observe long-term results.

We know so little about immune system function at different ages that we should not stand pat on the basis of studies that can find no harm in the immunization programs. We have epidemics of obesity, cancer, and heart disease. Obesity is a marker of dietary excesses and deficiencies that contribute to the development of these disorders. Nutritional factors have a profound effect on immune function. Is it too big of a step to say that many mothers in this culture have not endowed their newborns with the best immune function? We do not know when the individual infant has its immune system in gear, ready for the assault of multiple immunizations. We measure antibody response to individual antigens when they are given at the same time as others, but we know little else about the interactions that can affect other aspects of the immune system.

In nutrition, we deal with the "mole hills," such as the prevention of spina bifida (a serious but rare condition) with folic acid intake—information that is of little value in a quick well-child check—and ignore the "mountains," the obesity that points to the need to communicate the value of an understanding of total nutrition.

If I sound like an advocate of the good ol' days, I am. But I am realistic enough to know that we cannot completely go back. In the first place, we cannot find the time in an insurance-ordered system, and if we could, who is going to reimburse the physician for his time and experience? Nor can we reverse the medicine-and-tests-oriented trend that is so revered. We do need to interject more clinical know-how and slow the prescription writing. Don't throw away what works from a past era. Remember that "the new" can have glitches.

Today, with widespread and easy access to the Internet, we can all tap into a plethora of information which can include nutrition and medicine studies. Many of the postings on either side need to be scrutinized because of the bias of those striving for financial gain. Few of us have the background of years of analyzing the contents of these articles to feel confident that they represent "truth" or that they are just good for promoting sales. As a young, busy physician, I trusted what my authority, the American Academy of Pediatrics, published in its journal. Fortunately, in the early days of my practice, there was little use of medicines in pediatrics and many articles were written by experts who are now considered "nutrition giants." I had no need to question an article's validity until, somehow, a battle between "medicine" and "nutrition" began. Pediatric "medical disorders" seemed to be concocted in order to create a need for a financially rewarding pharmaceutical remedy.

A light bulb didn't suddenly turn on, but gradually I realized there was a lot of phoniness in the process of posting information. Big

Pharma's influence is considerable. They have been in the position of submitting their own studies for acceptance of a new drug by the Food and Drug Administration (FDA). Recently, whistle-blowers who uncovered the fact that some of the studies were fraudulent have been successful in presenting cases to the courts. A recent case involved pharmaceutical representatives (detail men), who advised doctor clients to prescribe medicines for children (even very young children), even though the drugs had not been approved by the FDA for use in children. This practice met with full approval from company executives. The fine of 3 *billion* dollars certainly got their attention, and should get the attention of all consumers. How can that industry be trusted? Because of the powerful lure of financial gain, even nutrition studies were sometimes corrupted. Bad as that is, the side effects of taking an overly hyped nutrition supplement will never equal the potentially very dangerous side effects of a drug. So how does one filter out the "bad" and know the "good"? It can only be done by turning to trustworthy, unbiased researchers. Orthomolecular medicine can put you on the right track through the "suggested reading" and "references" in this book. These will get you to the point to where you can make your own tailor-made judgment call.

Helen Saul Case, in her book, *The Vitamin Cure for Women's Health Problems*, suggests that there are times you need to go to your doctor to get an accurate diagnosis. You can hope that he or she will be nutrition-oriented and discuss vitamin therapy for the ailment at hand. If not, accept the prescription, then do your homework. Unless the doctor convinces you that this is a medical emergency and that it is imperative that you fill the prescription, you might give the vitamin therapy a fair trial. If you get better, continue. If not, consider filling the prescription. These "prescribe first" practices are being pushed down into the toddler age group. Very dangerous, indeed.

In the United States the political battle over nationalized "health care" has been, in reality, only about insurance care. Who is going to pay the premiums, and how are they going to do it? There has been absolutely no talk about health. Neither side offers anything resembling healthy thinking. Drugs modify sickness. They are not the way of achieving good health. This book gives concrete examples of cost savings that seem to be ignored by politicians. Realizing that throughout the "civilized" world basic health measures are being put aside in favor of medicines, leads me to tears.

And now the FDA is putting injectable vitamin C and injectable B vitamins into the *drug* category. In our opinion, their ultimate agenda is to make all vitamin supplements require a prescription. It is time to speak up and speak out.

APPENDIX 1

SEVEN DAYS OF LACTO-VEGETARIAN MENU FOR A WEANED BABY

very time my children and I (AWS) went to dinner at my parents' house, my mother would invariably say, "We don't know what to feed you people!" "You people" refers in this case to a family that did not eat meat, but did eat pretty much everything else. So I would always answer with the same phrase: "Mom, prepare and serve whatever you wish to, and we will choose from what you set out. No problem."

It's not that difficult to raise meatless-diet kids, but in my opinion, it is very difficult to raise healthy, totally vegetarian (vegan) children. I would go so far as to recommend against raising kids without dairy foods and eggs. Cheese, yogurt, and eggs are super-good foods for little kids (big ones, too). There are few eggs in this menu plan, however. Looking back, I would lean towards offering some egg yolk (easiest to digest, and tastiest) every day for a baby. Egg white is fine too: a good protein source, but in my opinion, better for "older babies."

Note: Unless otherwise stated, give the child as much as they desire of the foods listed below.

MONDAY

Breakfast

Wheatena or other whole-grain
  hot cereal

Fruit

$1/4$ of a chewable vitamin C 500
  mg tablet (125 mg) is what
  we gave our toddlers. Infants,
  half of that ($1/8$ tablet, about
  60 mg) crushed to a fine
  powder and put in applesauce
  or similar food.

$1/3$ teaspoon liquid multiple
  vitamin

Lunch

Beans

Corn

Squash or pumpkin

Cottage cheese

$1/4$ of a chewable C 500 mg
  tablet, crushed into a fine
  powder

$1/3$ teaspoon liquid multiple
  vitamin

Supper

Cottage cheese or yogurt

Puffed wheat (no milk needed;
  use a few at a time as a
  finger-food)

One slice whole-wheat bread
  with butter

Fruit

$1/4$ of a chewable C 500 mg
  tablet

TUESDAY

Breakfast

Oatmeal or other whole-grain
  hot cereal

Fruit

$1/4$ chewable C 500 mg tablet

$1/3$ teaspoon liquid multiple
  vitamin

Lunch

Peas (or other green vegetable)

Corn

Squash or pumpkin

Cottage cheese

$1/4$ chewable C 500 mg tablet

$1/3$ teaspoon liquid multiple
  vitamin

Supper

Cottage cheese

Pumpkin bread (two slices),
  or

Whole-grain muffins (one or
  two), or

Whole-wheat bread with
  butter

Fruit

$1/4$ of a chewable C 500 mg
  tablet

WEDNESDAY

Breakfast

Oatmeal cereal or other whole-grain hot cereal

Fruit

$1/4$ chewable C 500 mg tablet

$1/3$ teaspoon liquid multiple vitamin

Lunch

Beans

Corn

Squash or pumpkin

Cottage vheese

$1/4$ chewable C 500 mg tablet

$1/3$ teaspoon liquid multiple vitamin

Supper

Poached egg on whole-wheat toast

Juice

Ice cream (a natural-ingredients brand)

$1/4$ of a chewable C 500 mg tablet

THURSDAY

Breakfast

Oatmeal

Fruit

$1/4$ chewable C 500 mg tablet

$1/3$ teaspoon liquid multiple vitamin

Lunch

Peas or other green vegetable

Corn

Squash or pumpkin

Cottage cheese

$1/4$ chewable C 500 mg tablet

$1/3$ teaspoon liquid multiple vitamin

Supper

Cottage cheese

Puffed wheat, or

Whole-wheat bread with butter

Fruit

$1/4$ of a chewable C 500 mg tablet

MAKE CHEW-ABLES DO-ABLE

Toddlers usually, and infants for certain, need their chewable vitamin C crushed into a powder before you give it to them. Exactly when a child is old enough to chew a tablet will vary. Kids tend to let you know these things, but as you sit in the big chair, you need to observe and decide when the time is right. When in doubt, powder it out.

FRIDAY

Breakfast

Wheatena or other whole-grain hot cereal

Fruit

1/4 chewable C 500 mg tablet

1/3 teaspoon liquid multiple vitamin

Lunch

Beans

Corn

Squash or pumpkin

Cottage cheese or yogurt

1/4 chewable C 500 mg tablet

1/3 teaspoon liquid multiple vitamin

Supper

French toast (whole-grain bread, with butter and pure maple syrup or comb honey)

Fruit

1/4 of a chewable C 500 mg tablet

SATURDAY

Breakfast

Oatmeal

Fruit

1/4 chewable C 500 mg tablet

1/3 teaspoon liquid multiple vitamin

Lunch

Peas or other green vegetable

Corn

Squash

Cottage cheese or yogurt

1/4 chewable C 500 mg tablet

1/3 teaspoon liquid multiple vitamin

Supper

Poached egg on whole-wheat toast (one slice, with butter)

Juice

Ice cream (any natural brand)

1/4 of a chewable C 500 mg tablet

SUNDAY

Breakfast

Oatmeal cereal or other whole-
grain hot cereal

Fruit

$1/4$ chewable C 500 mg tablet

$1/3$ teaspoon liquid multiple
vitamin

Lunch

Beans

Corn

Squash or pumpkin

Cottage cheese

$1/4$ chewable C 500 mg tablet

$1/3$ teaspoon liquid multiple
vitamin

Supper

Cottage cheese or yogurt

Pumpkin bread, or

Whole-grain muffin
(homemade, low sugar)

Whole-wheat bread with butter

Fruit

$1/4$ of a chewable C 500 mg
tablet

This is pretty much the exact diet we raised our two children with, from the time they first showed interest in solid food up until age two or so. It is a simple diet, but quite high in protein. Corn, beans, and squash (or pumpkin) together form a complete protein equal to that in meats. Eggs, cottage cheese, and dairy products in general are complete proteins, also. We would frequently add an egg to any given meal if the child was especially hungry, in a growth spurt (which was *often!*) for more filling, stick-to-the-ribs satiety.

If children are hungry, feed them all they want . . . of good food only. That is the trick: You select; they choose. Providing the illusion of choice is always a good trick to know. Here it is as applied to mealtime: only buy healthy food; only have good food in the house; serve only good food. Sounds redundantly simplistic, but try it and see.

We recommend only whole-grain breads, preferably homemade when possible. Whole grains are surprisingly high in protein. If your baby has issues with wheat, or just a sensitive digestion, try non-wheat alternatives available at any health food store and most supermarkets. Any whole-grain flour of your choice an be used to make breads and muffins. And don't forget that French toast, pancakes, and waffles are unbelievably yummy to little children. Adults, too.

You will notice that most breakfasts and suppers call for fruit. This keeps the baby's bowel habits regular and easy. Fruit should be fresh whenever possible and served with skins peeled off and the fruit cut into small pieces. Canned fruits may be used, but should be juice-packed as opposed to syrup packed. You can use syrup-packed fruit if you rinse the fruit in a glass container before serving it. Do not rinse the fruit in the can or it will taste like the can.

Raw foods, such as grated vegetables, sprouted beans, and sprouted grains should be encouraged as soon as a child can eat them easily. Mash anything with a fork to make it easier to eat, or use a hand baby-food grinder or blender. Corn and beans are best mashed up for easier diges-tion in the early months before your baby can or will chew thoroughly.

We gave our babies a small bit of vitamin C with *every meal,* and with every nursing or snack. Powder one-fourth of a chewable 500 mg vitamin C tablet between two spoons and slip it into the child's fruit or unsweetened juice. (This is important, and that is why we are repeating it.)

You probably noticed that beverages in general and "milk" in par-ticular are not included in this schedule. Water, natural unsweetened fruit juice, and vegetable juice are all good. If there are cheeses in the diet, you really do not need fluid milk. Consider milk to be optional, not essential.

This diet example is in no way meant to replace your pediatrician, whom you should see when necessary. This diet may, however, help rel-egate your doctor to the role of the repairman you never need. That's fine! Our children have never had an antibiotic in their entire lives, and they are now in college. That is why we recommend the vitamin C sup-plement with every meal, and why we raised them on a meatless menu, like this one.

By far the best way to get a little one to eat right is for the parents to eat right. Monkey-see monkey-do is not always a bad thing. Lions actively teach their cubs to hunt. We can teach our children to eat right before they even know there is a choice to eat wrong. It is not neces-sarily an active process. Parents set an example whether they wish to or not. Nobel laureate Albert Schweitzer, M.D., said, "Not only is example the best way to teach, it is the only way."

If you do not want to go for the "full Monty" of a raw-food vegetarian diet, that just do a regular no-junk-food, meatless diet and load up on foods that really do need cooking: the legumes. Peas, beans, and lentils are high in fiber, cheap, and filling. They are also high in the dieter's friend, tryptophan, the feel-good amino acid mentioned above.

Be sure to eat your squash, too. People who complain that vegetarian eating does not satisfy their hunger are doing it wrong. Follow the ways of the Native Americans and always invite all of the Three Sisters to your dinner table: grain, legumes, and squash. If you eat a lot of just one or two parts of this triad, you will likely still have the after-dinner munchies. When you have roughly equal servings of grain, beans, and squash at each meal, you prepare yourself for entry into a whole different between-meal world: a world in which you are happy and the cravings are gone.

Should you feel a bit tenuous about crafting the lacto-ovo-veggie child, here follows is a second opinion from Dr. Campbell:

My (RKC) feeling is that somehow or other, early in life, most infants "get by"(just by) if parents follow conventional advice—even the substandard RDAs. But this is the perfect time to establish good eating patterns that can be optimized with the toddler, on up. Certainly, pay attention to the superiority of nursing first. "Near-vegetarian babies," critics might say, sounds "off the wall." Not so, when experience shows that it works and is safe. This menu provides good information for those that predominately go "veggie" —describing how to get complete proteins from the right combinations. A "lacto-ovo" diet assures adequate B_{12} and zinc intake. I worry about those on a strict, no-dairy or egg vegetarian (vegan) diet. Remember that we need to always be age-appropriate; we need to avoid irritating an infant's bowel with chunks of fiber that are too large. The simple, effective way to resolve this is to use a blender for fruits, and also blending or hand-foodmill-grinding cooked as well as raw vegetables. Add foods one at a time to check them out and see how your child responds to them.

I don't consider myself as a passive parent, but I was not as rigorous as Dr. Saul was in my approach to nutrition for infants and toddlers. Much of the reason being my ignorance, at that time, about optimal nutrition and listening only to the advice of the learned men in the American Academy of Pediatrics. We, as new parents, were still of a culture that ate *real* food—the foods we were raised on—that seemed to work for us. There was the added advantage of growing up in Southern California where fresh fruits and vegetables were available and cheap. (Would you believe that beautiful cabbage, raised by Japanese Americans, cost the outrageous price of two heads for a nickel?)

Meat didn't come from grain- and drug-fattened feedlot cattle but from nearby meat distributors of grass-fed, antibiotic-free animals. Sugar-coated cold cereals were nonexistent. Children were offered a soda as a treat, only on rare occasions. Today, we eat far too much meat, corrupted processed foods, and down an amazing quantity of sugar. (More on this topic is in the chapter on feeding).

I am certain that Dr. Saul's suggested diet menu would have tremendous benefits. It would be the opposite of today's regular fare. I am not sure if we had the chance to repeat raising our children that we would have been as disciplined. Let's find the core of this menu and apply it. We can trim the edges without cutting into the "meat" of it. A little safe, organic meat is okay. Think of the ideally healthy diet for us as adults and progress toward that, while keeping in mind what the digestive tract limitations of infancy and early childhood dictate. Be conscious of the particle size of foods, especially of fibrous (indigestible) fruits and vegetables. The infant intestinal tract was designed to accommodate the ultimate nonfibrous food—breast milk. The transition to "people's foods" should be made cautiously. There are big individual differences in the time of a successful transition. Judge by checking the stools for chunks of undigested food or for mucus that represent an irritated bowel (the latter is usually accompanied by some signs of a bellyache).

A Feeding Plan
for a Healthy Baby

BY HELEN SAUL CASE

Helen is AWS' daughter, who was raised as described above. She is now a parent herself, and has kindly contributed her views.

The way I was raised, it was pretty much a no-brainer decision. When our daughter was born, my husband and I knew she would be breast-fed, and thankfully that was a success. We knew we would feed her the best possible diet. She nursed for just over a year, and as she grew hungrier, we would give her organic fruits and grains in addition to breast milk. Once she was weaned, we continued giving her vegetable and fruit purees and then soft or easily dissolvable foods like chunks of fruit, cereals, and cooked eggs. Now she can chew pretty well, and items like apple pieces and toast go down without any trouble. She's now about a year and a half old. Below outlines many of her food choices, all which have been a success.

Organic egg on organic whole-wheat toast with organic butter (and occasionally organic ketchup) and French toast

Watermelon, honeydew, and cantaloupe

Tofu (prepared with some flavor like garlic)

Cheese: cheddar, Munster, mozzarella, whatever!

Organic whole milk yogurt

Natural peanut butter on organic crackers, grahams, or whole-wheat toast

Sweet potato or regular potato and sour cream

Cooked eel and crab with avocado and brown rice (from our sushi dishes)

Prunes: puréed and when she was older, cut-up whole prunes: These get just about anything else down. I put prunes on the front of the spoon, and then whatever else I want her to eat on the back and down it goes. Yay, prunes!

Peas or anything else she won't eat, equally mixed with Panaek paler (an Indian spinach dish). This is a salty item, so I always cut it with unsalted baby food. In fact, she is a fan of much of the Indian food at your standard buffet. This may be because I ate a lot of spicy foods while pregnant . . .

The Three Sisters: squash, corn, and beans (refried works, too)

Tomatoes, and if I can't find organic, I just wash the tomatoes with soap and water or rely on neighbors that have gardens and don't use pesticides.

Cucumbers, peeled

Organic strawberries, peaches, pears, grapes, apples (or applesauce), blueberries, and bananas

Organic pasta blended with organic sauce, garlic, and cheese

Organic oat O's cereal

Organic rice puffs (for stroller snacks)

Cooked organic carrots, onions (in homemade soup)

While she isn't on a strict vegetarian diet, I feel she is getting plenty of nutrition from other nonmeat foods. If she has meat, it is a rare occurrence, and I make sure it is organic too.

Convenient Foods

There is quite a selection of organic baby foods on the market, even those in convenient little pouches instead of jars. She can just suck some right out of the container! These are great for when we travel and visit, and are handy in a pinch at home or to keep her happy on a long grocery trip where everything she points to is "Nana! Nana!" including the bananas. It's nice to see my child pointing to tomatoes, bananas, grapes hoping for handouts instead of pointing at items in the cookie aisle. Frankly, we haven't even been down that aisle.

Food Combinations

Here are some of the organic store-bought pouch, jar, and packet combinations she likes. I tend to buy ones that have a mix of a fruit and vegetable, rather than fruit alone. (She has no trouble eating yummy sweet fruit. It is harder to get spinach, peas or broccoli down.)

Butternut squash macaroni and cheese

Broccoli and apple

Peaches, pumpkin, and grain

Sweet potatoes and beans or with corn and apple

Sweet potatoes, pumpkin, and fruit

Banana and squash

Lentils and tomatoes

Squash, carrots, apples, and prunes

Carrots and apples with or without mango

Apples, blueberries, and spinach

Spinach, peas, and pear

Yogurt, fruit, and grains

Fruit-only combinations like strawberry apple, peach banana, or apple blackberry (for treats)

Fruit and grain combinations like banana and brown rice or prunes and oatmeal

Beverages

We keep it simple here. Most of the time she is drinking water or milk. Occasionally I slip in some fruit juice, but this is rare. I prefer she get her fruit straight from the source. Carrot juice is a great addition to mix it up.

Organic milk

Fresh homemade sweet, organic carrot juice or store bought

Water

Watered down yogurt or whole milk kefir

Rarely: orange juice or lemonade watered down 1 part juice/lemonade to 3 parts water

Vitamins

Our daughter also gets her vitamins. Most days, she gets a dose of a children's liquid multivitamin at breakfast in the morning, and then a dose of liquid vitamin C at each of the next two meals. Since liquid C loses potency over time, I mix in about one to two teaspoons of buffered vitamin C in the form of calcium ascorbate into a four ounce jar of liquid every five days or so. I reduce how much vitamin C I add as the liquid dwindles. It is not an exact science, but it doesn't need to be. I figure she gets somewhere around 100–250 mg of C in each dose. When she is tooting away, I know she's had enough. Before vaccinations, she gets more C. After vaccinations, I give her even more. She will get vitamin C every one and a half to two hours until she gets gassy.

Managing Friends, Family, and Food

Not everyone has a fridge stocked with organic produce. This was especially true when Connie would visit friends and family. She would often be more interested in the food choices they had than what was packed in her lunch bag. I can't blame her, really. I have always found the contents of other people's refrigerators to be more exciting than my own.

I knew I couldn't always monitor what she ate, so I set down some basic ground rules for friends and family about what she can and cannot have: no artificial sweeteners, no sugar before bed, and *very* limited sugar during the day (for example, a bite of ice cream is okay, but not a bowl full), no meat, and no artificially colored anything.

I encourage them to wash grapes and other such foods with soap and water, as water alone does not remove pesticides, but I know this rarely happens. (Great Grandma looked at me like I was nuts, and then gave her a "washed" grape anyway.) In fact, most folks look at me like I'm crazy when I even suggest using soap too. So, if I'm concerned that I will be up against some tough opposition, I just pack the organic item I want her to have, and if she wants grapes, oh, look! We just happen to have some packed and ready to eat.

Another great example is yogurt. Many varieties found in folks' fridges are "light" and packed with artificial colors, fake sweeteners, and indigestible fillers like modified food starch. So, I pack organic yogurt for her too, with some fruit to mix in to make it appetizing. This way, it's pretty clear what I intend for her to eat. The rest of course, is up to her caregiver at the time.

Because I am seen as protective when it comes to her food choices, announcing that while I was away she was given white bread (gasp!) and butter is thought to bother me. I act slightly annoyed, and then smile to myself. If that's the worst she is given, I think we are all set.

I value the time I get to spend alone with my hubby, and I value the time my daughter gets to spend with her extended family and our friends. I accept that some foods she will get (now and forever . . . just wait until she rides a bus to school) are not always going to contain optimum levels of nutrition. We just make a point to feed her the best we can whenever we can. This has worked out well so far.

Shock Your Pediatrician

The other day I shocked my pediatrician who looked at my year-and-a-half-old daughter's chart and said, "Wow! She's only in here for wellness visits and vaccines!"

I smiled.

She continued, "You should have seen the chart on the last child I met with. There was always something wrong!"

Perhaps this speaks for itself.

APPENDIX 3

VITAMIN C PREVENTS VACCINATION SIDE EFFECTS; INCREASES EFFECTIVENESS

by Thomas E Levy, MD, JD

(OMNS, Feb 14, 2012) The routine administration of vaccinations continues to be a subject of controversy in the United States, as well as throughout the world. Parents who want the best for their babies and children continue to be faced with decisions that they fear could harm their children if made incorrectly. The controversy over the potential harm of vaccinating, or of not vaccinating, will not be resolved to the satisfaction of all parties anytime soon, if ever. This brief report aims to offer some practical information to pediatricians and parents alike who want the best long-term health for their patients and children, regardless of their sentiments on the topic of vaccination in general.

While there seems to be a great deal of controversy over how frequently a vaccination might result in a negative outcome, there is little controversy that at least some of the time vaccines do cause damage. The question that then emerges is whether something can be done to minimize, if not eliminate, the infliction of such damage, however infrequently it may occur.

Causes of Vaccination Side Effects

When vaccines do have side effects and adverse reactions, these outcomes are often categorized as resulting from allergic reactions or the result of a negative interaction with compromised immune systems. While either of these types of reactions can be avoided subsequently when there is a history of a bad reaction having occurred at least once in the past as a result of a vaccination, it is vital to try to avoid encountering a negative outcome from occurring the first time vaccines are administered.

Due to the fact that all toxins, toxic effects, substantial allergic reactions, and induced immune compromise have the final common denominator of causing and/or resulting in the oxidation of vital biomolecules, the antioxidant vitamin C has proven to be the ultimate nonspecific antidote to whatever toxin or excess oxidative stress might be present. While there is also a great deal of dispute over the inherent toxicity of the antigens that many vaccines present to the immune systems of those vaccinated, there is no question, for example, that thimerosal, a mercury-containing preservative, is highly toxic when present in significant amounts. This then begs the question: Rather than argue whether there is an infinitesimal, minimal, moderate, or significant amount of toxicity associated with the amounts of thimerosal or other potentially toxic components presently being used in vaccines, why not just neutralize whatever toxicity is present as completely and definitively as possible?

Vitamin C is a Potent Antitoxin

In addition to its general antitoxin properties (Levy, 2002), vitamin C has been demonstrated to be highly effective in neutralizing the toxic nature of mercury in all of its chemical forms. In animal studies, vitamin C can prevent the death of animals given otherwise fatal doses of mercury chloride (Mokranjac and Petrovic, 1964). Having vitamin C on board prior to mercury exposure was able to prevent the kidney damage the mercury otherwise typically caused (Carroll, et al., 1965). Vitamin C also blocked the fatal effect of mercury cyanide (Vauthey, 1951). Even the very highly toxic organic forms of mercury have been shown to be effectively detoxified by vitamin C (Gage, 1975).

Vitamin C Improves Vaccine Effectiveness

By potential toxicity considerations alone, then, there would seem to be no good reason not to pre- and post-medicate an infant or child with some amount of vitamin C to minimize or block the toxicity that might significantly affect a few. However, there is another compelling reason to make vitamin C an integral part of any vaccination protocol: Vitamin C has been documented to augment the antibody response of the immune system (Prinz et al., 1977; Vallance, 1977; Prinz et al., 1980; Feigen et al., 1982; Li and Lovell, 1985; Amakye-Anim et al., 2000; Wu et al., 2000; Lauridsen and Jensen, 2005; Azad et al., 2007). As the goal of any vaccination is to stimulate a maximal antibody response to the antigens of the vaccine while causing minimal to no toxic damage to the most sensitive of vaccine recipients, there would appear to be no medically sound reason not to make vitamin C a part of all vaccination protocols. Except in individuals with established, significant renal insufficiency, vitamin C is arguably the safest of all nutrients that can be given, especially in the amounts discussed below. Unlike virtually all prescription drugs and some supplements, vitamin C has never been found to have any dosage level above which it can be expected to demonstrate any toxicity.

Vitamin C Reduces Mortality in Vaccinated Infants and Children

Kalokerinos (1974) demonstrated repeatedly and quite conclusively that Aboriginal infants and children, a group with an unusually high death rate after vaccinations, were almost completely protected from this outcome by dosing them with vitamin C before and after vaccinations. The reason articulated for the high death rate was the exceptionally poor and near-scurvy-inducing (vitamin C-depleted) diet that was common in the Aboriginal culture. This also demonstrates that with the better nutrition in the United States and elsewhere in the world, the suggested doses of vitamin C should give an absolute protection against death (essentially a toxin-induced acute scurvy) and almost absolute protection against lesser toxic outcomes from any vaccinations administered. Certainly, there appears to be no logical reason not to give a nontoxic substance known to neutralize toxicity and stimulate antibody production, which is the whole point of vaccine administration.

Dosage Information for Pediatricians and Parents

Practically speaking, then, how should the pediatrician or parent proceed? For optimal antibody stimulation and toxin protection, it would be best to dose for three to five days before the shot(s) and to continue for at least two to three days following the shot. When dealing with infants and very young children, administering a 1,000 mg dose of liposome-encapsulated vitamin C would be both easiest and best, as the gel-like nature of this form of vitamin C allows a ready mixture into yogurt or any other palatable food, and the complete proximal absorption of the liposomes would avoid any possible loose stools or other possible undesirable bowel effects.

Vitamin C as sodium ascorbate powder will also work well. Infants under 10 pounds can take 500 mg daily in some fruit juice, while babies between 10 and 20 pounds could take anywhere from 500 mg to 1,000 mg total per day, in divided doses. Older children can take 1,000 mg daily per year of life (5,000 mg for a 5 year-old child, for example, in divided doses). If sodium must be avoided, calcium ascorbate is well-tolerated and, like sodium ascorbate, is non-acidic. Some but not all children's chewable vitamins are made with calcium ascorbate. Be sure to read the label. Giving vitamin C in divided doses, all through the day, improves absorption and improves tolerance. As children get older, they can more easily handle the ascorbic acid form of vitamin C, especially if given with meals. For any child showing significant bowel sensitivity, either use liposome-encapsulated vitamin C, or the amount of regular vitamin C can just be appropriately decreased to an easily tolerated amount.

Very similar considerations exist for older individuals receiving any of a number of vaccinations for preventing infection, such as the yearly flu shots. When there is really no urgency, and there rarely is, such individuals should supplement with vitamin C for several weeks before and several weeks after, if at all possible.

Even taking a one-time dose of vitamin C in the dosage range suggested above directly before the injections can still have a significant toxin-neutralizing and antibody-stimulating effect. It's just that an even better likelihood of having a positive outcome results from extending the pre- and post-dosing periods of time.

(Reprinted with permission. Thomas Levy, MD, JD is a board-certified cardiologist and admitted to the bar in Colorado and the District of Colombia. He is the author of several books on vitamin C as well as numerous articles. A vitamin C lecture by Dr. Levy may be viewed at: http://www.youtube.com/watch?v=k0GC9Fq8lfg)

References

Amakye-Anim, J., T. Lin, P. Hester, et al. (2000) Ascorbic acid supplementation improved antibody response to infectious bursal disease vaccination in chickens. *Poultry Science* 79:680–688

Azad, I., J. Dayal, M. Poornima, and S. Ali (2007) Supra dietary levels of vitamins C and E enhance antibody production and immune memory in juvenile milkfish, *Chanos chanos* (Forsskal) to formalin-killed *Vibrio vulnificus*. *Fish & Shellfish Immunology* 23:154–163

Carroll, R., K. Kovacs, and E. Tapp (1965) Protection against mercuric chloride poisoning of the rat kidney. *Arzneimittelforschung* 15:1361–1363

Feigen, G., B. Smith, C. Dix, et al. (1982) Enhancement of antibody production and protection against systemic anaphylaxis by large doses of vitamin C. *Research Communications in Chemical Pathology and Pharmacology* 38:313–333

Gage, J. (1975) Mechanisms for the biodegradation of organic mercury compounds: the actions of ascorbate and of soluble proteins. *Toxicology and Applied Pharmacology* 32:225–238

Kalokerinos, A. (1974) *Every Second Child*. New Canaan, CT: Keats Publishing, Inc.

Lauridsen, C. and S. Jensen (2005) Influence of supplementation of all-rac-alpha-tocopheryl acetate preweaning and vitamin C postweaning on alpha-tocopherol and immune responses in piglets. *Journal of Animal Science* 83:1274–1286

Levy, T. (2004) *Curing the Incurable. Vitamin C, Infectious Diseases, and Toxins*. Henderson, NV: MedFox Publishing

Li, Y. and R. Lovell (1985) Elevated levels of dietary ascorbic acid increase immune responses in channel catfish. *The Journal of Nutrition* 115:123–131

Mokranjac, M. and C. Petrovic (1964) Vitamin C as an antidote in poisoning by fatal doses of mercury. *Comptes Rendus Hebdomadaires des Seances de l'Academie des Sciences* 258:1341–1342

Prinz, W., R. Bortz, B. Bregin, and M. Hersch (1977) The effect of ascorbic acid supplementation on some parameters of the human immunological defence system. *International Journal for Vitamin and Nutrition Research* 47:248–257

Prinz, W., J. Bloch, G., G. Gilich, and G. Mitchell (1980) A systematic study of the effect of vitamin C supplementation on the humoral immune response in ascorbate-dependent mammals. I. The antibody response to sheep red blood cells (a T-dependent antigen) in guinea pigs. *International Journal for Vitamin and Nutrition Research* 50:294–300

Vallance, S. (1977) Relationships between ascorbic acid and serum proteins of the immune system. *British Medical Journal* 2:437–438

Vauthey, M. (1951) Protective effect of vitamin C against poisons. *Praxis (Bern)* 40:284–286

Wu, C., T. Dorairajan, and T. Lin (2000) Effect of ascorbic acid supplementation on the immune response of chickens vaccinated and challenged with infectious bursal disease virus. *Veterinary Immunology and Immunopathology* 74:145–152

RECOMMENDED
READING

Clarke, J. H. *The Prescriber.* 4th Edition. Essex, UK: C. W. Daniel Co., 1972.

Coulter, H. L. *Homeopathic Science and Modern Medicine: The Physics of Healing with Microdoses.* Richmond, CA: North Atlantic Books, 1981.

Ginott, H. G. *Between Parent and Child: The Bestselling Classic that Revolutionized Parent-Child Communication.* New York: Three Rivers Press, 2003.

Ginott, H. G. *Between Parent and Teenager.* New York: Macmillan, 1969.

Ginott, H. G. *Teacher and Child: A Book for Parents and Teachers.* New York: Maxwell Macmillian International, 1993.

Hickey, S., A. W. Saul. *Vitamin C: The Real Story.* Laguna Beach, CA: Basic Health, 2008.

Landwehr, R. "The Origin of the 42-Year Stonewall of Vitamin C." *J Orthomolecular Med* 6(2) (1991):99–103. Available online at http://orthomolecular.org/library/jom/1991/pdf/1991-v06n02-p099.pdf (accessed April 2013)

Levy, T. E. *Vitamin C, Infectious Diseases, and Toxins: Curing the Incurable.* Philadelphia, PA: Xlibris Corporation, 2002, 52–53. Reviewed in *J Orthomolecular Med* 18(2) 2003:117–118.

Miller, F. "Dr. Klenner Urges Taking Vitamins in Huge Doses." *Greensboro Daily News* Dec 13, 1977, A8-A10.

Pollan, M. *In Defense of Food: An Eater's Manifesto.* New York: Penguin Press, 2008.

Saul, A. W. "The Pioneering Work of William J. McCormick, M.D." *J Orthomolecular Med,* 18(2) 2003:93–96. Available online at: http://www.doctoryourself.com/mccormick.html (accessed Oct 2012).

Saul, A. W. "Taking the cure: Claus Washington Jungeblut, M.D.: Polio Pioneer; Ascorbate Advocate." *J Orthomolecular Med* 21(2) 2006:102–106. Available online at http://www.doctoryourself.com/jungeblut.html (accessed Oct 2012).

Schlosser, E. *Fast Food Nation: The Dark Side of the All-American Meal.* Boston, MA: Houghton Mifflin, 2001.

Smith, L. H. *Clinical Guide to the Use of Vitamin C: The Clinical Experiences of Frederick R. Klenner, M.D.* Portland, OR: Life Sciences Press, 1988. Adapted from: *Vitamin C as a Fundamental Medicine: Abstracts of Dr. Frederick R. Klenner, M.D.'s Published and Unpublished Work.* Reprinted 1991. Available online at http://www.whale.to/a/smith_b.html (accessed April 2013).

Stone, I. *The Healing Factor: Vitamin C Against Disease.* NY: Grosset & Dunlap, 1972; 191–192. Available online at: http://vitamincfoundation.org/stone/ (accessed Oct 2012).

A Brief Listing of Titles by Frederick R. Klenner

If you are really keen on this subject, you will discover that only two of Dr. Frederick R. Klenner's many papers are currently indexed by MEDLINE. Yes, unfortunately, it is true. The U.S. National Library of Medicine, the world's largest medical library, indexes nothing whatsoever written by Klenner after 1952, when he published primarily in the *Tri-State Medical Journal*.

Klenner, F. R. "Case History: The Black Widow Spider." *Tri-State Med J* (Dec 1957)

Klenner, F. R. "Case History: Cure of a 4-Year Old Child Bitten by a Mature Highland Moccasin with Vitamin C." *Tri-State Med J* (Jul 1954). Author's note: The Highland Moccasin, a viper, is also known as the copperhead.

Klenner, F. R. "A Critical Analysis of the Francis Report Concerning the 1954 Poliomyelitis Vaccine Program." *Tri-State Med J* (Jun 1955).

Klenner, F. R. "Encephalitis as a sequelae of the pneumonias." *Tri-State Med J* (Feb 1960):7–11.

Klenner, F. R. "The Folly in the Continued Use of a Killed Polio Virus Vaccine." *Tri-State Med J* (Feb 1959):1–8.

Klenner, F. R. "The History of Lockjaw." *Tri-State Med J* (Jun 1954).

Klenner, F. R. "An Insidious Virus." *Tri-State Med J* (Jun 1957).

Klenner, F. R. "Massive Doses of Vitamin C and the Virus Diseases." *Southern Med Surg* 13(4) (Apr 1951):101–107. Available online at http://www.whale.to/a/klenner1951ds.html (accessed April 2013). This paper is sometimes erroneously cited as 103(4).

Klenner, F. R. "A New Office Procedure for the Determination of Plasma Levels for Ascorbic Acid." *Tri-State Medical J* (Feb 1956):26–28.

Klenner, F. R. "Observations on the Dose and Administration of Ascorbic Acid When Employed Beyond the Range of a Vitamin in Human Pathology." *J Appl Nutr* 23(3–4) (Winter 1971). Available online at: http://www.orthomed.com/klenner.htm and http://www.doctoryourself.com/klennerpaper.html (accessed Oct 2012).

Klenner, F. R. "Poliomyelitis: Case Histories." *Tri-State Med J* (Sep 1956):28–31.

Klenner, F. R. "Poliomyelitis Vaccine: Brodie vs. Salk." *Tri-State Med J* (Jul 1955).

Klenner, F. R. "The Role of Ascorbic Acid in Therapeutics." (Letter) *Tri-State Med J* (Nov 1955):34.

Klenner, F. R. "Recent Discoveries in the Treatment of Lockjaw with Vitamin C and Tolserol." *Tri-State Med J* (Jul 1954).

Klenner, F. R. "Significance of High Daily Intake of Ascorbic Acid in Preventive Medicine." *J Int Acad Prev Med* 1(1) (Spring 1974):45–69. Also in: Williams, R. J., D. K. Kalita, editors. *A Physician's Handbook on Orthomolecular Medicine*. 3rd ed. New York: Pergamon Press, 1977: 51–59.

Klenner, F. R. "The Treatment of Poliomyelitis and Other Virus Diseases with Vitamin C." *Southern Med Surg* 111(7) (Jul 1949):209–214. Available online at http://www.whale.to/v/c/klenner3.html (accessed April 2013).

Klenner, F. R. "A Treatment of Trichinosis with Massive Doses of Vitamin C and Para-Aminobenzoic Acid." *Tri-State Medical J* (Apr 1954).

Klenner, F. R. "The Use of Vitamin C as an Antibiotic." *J of Appl Nutr* 6 (1953):274–278. Available at http://whale.to/v/c/klenner1.html and at http://www.injectablevitaminc.com/images/Ch10.pdf (both accessed April 2013).

Klenner, F. R. "Virus Pneumonia and Its Treatment with Vitamin C." *Southern Med Surg* 110(2) (Feb1948):36–38, 46. Available online at http://www.whale.to/v/c/klenner2.html and at http://injectablevitaminc.com/images/Ch4.pdf (both accessed April 2013).

Klenner, F. R. "The Vitamin and Massage Treatment for Acute Poliomyelitis." *Southern Med Surg* 114(8) (aug 1952):194–7.

For More Information About:

Claus W. Jungeblut, M. D.

Saul, A. "Claus Washington Jungeblut, M.D.: Polio Pioneer; Ascorbate Advocate." *J Orthomolecular Med*, 21(2) (2006):102–106. http://www.doctoryourself.com/jungeblut.html (accessed Nov 2012).

Dr. Jungeblut's polio papers include:

Jungeblut, C. W. "Vitamin C Therapy and Prophylaxis in Experimental Poliomyelitis." *J Exp Med* 65(1) (Jan 1937):127–146.

Jungeblut, C. W. "Further Observations on Vitamin C Therapy in Experimental Poliomyelitis." *J Exper Med* 66(4) (Spe 30, 1937):459–477.

Jungeblut, C. W., R. R. Feiner. "Vitamin C Content of Monkey Tissues in Experimental Poliomyelitis." *J Exper Med* 66(4) (Sep 30, 1937):479–491.

Jungeblut, C. W. "A Further Contribution to Vitamin C Therapy in Experimental Poliomyelitis." *J Exper Med* 70(3) (Aug 31, 1939):315–332.

Jungeblut's research published in the *Journal of Experimental Medicine* is available for free access at http://www.jem.org/contents-by-date.0.shtml.

Frederick R. Klenner, M.D.

Saul, A. W. "Hidden in Plain Sight: The Pioneering Work of Frederick Robert Klenner, M.D." *J Orthomolecular Med* 22(1) (2007):31–38. http://www.doctoryourself.com/klennerbio.html (accessed Nov 2012). Also: http://orthomolecular.org/hof/2005/fklenner.html. (accessed Nov 2012).

William J. McCormick, M.D.

Saul, A. W. "The Pioneering Work of William J. McCormick, M.D." *J Orthomolecular Med* 18(2) (2003): reprinted with permission at http://www.doctoryourself.com/mccormick.html (accessed Nov 2012). Also: http://orthomolecular.org/hof/2004/wmccormick.html

Robert F. Cathcart III, M.D.

Biographical information can be found at: http://orthomolecular.org/hof/2008/cathcart.html (accessed Nov 2012).

Writings include:

Cathcart, R. F. "Vitamin C, Titrating to Bowel Tolerance, Anascorbemia, and Acute Induced Scurvy." *Med Hypotheses* 7 (1981): 1359–1376. http://www.doctoryourself .com/titration.html (accessed Nov 2012).

Cathcart, R. F. "Key Articles, 1975–2005." DoctorYourself.com. http://www .doctoryourself.com/biblio_cathcart.html (accessed Nov 2012).

Hugh D. Riordan, M.D.

Biographical information can be found at: http://orthomolecular.org/hof/2005/hriordan.html (accessed Nov 2012).

Writings include:

Riordan, H. D., X. Meng, J. Casciari, et al. "Intravenous Vitamin C is Selectively Toxic to Cancer Cells." *P Natl Acad Sci USA* Sep 12, 2005). A brief summary is available at http://orthomolecular.org/resources/omns/v01n09.shtml (accessed Nov 2012).

The Center for the Improvement of Human Functioning, International, Inc., Bio-Communications Research Institute. "Intravenous Ascorbate as a Chemotherapeutic and Biologic Response Modifying Agent." Reprinted with permission at: http://www.doctoryourself.com/riordan1.html (accessed Nov 2012).

"Hugh D. Riordan, M.D. Bibliography." DoctorYourself.com. http://www .doctoryourself.com/biblio_riordan.html (accessed Nov 2012).

REFERENCES

Chapter 1. How I Became a Parent and a Pediatrician

1. Campbell, R. K., A. W. Saul. *The Vitamin Cure for Children's Health Problems.* Laguna Beach, CA: Basic Health Publications, 2012.

Chapter 2. Immunizations

1. National Research Council. *DPT Vaccine and Chronic Nervous System Dysfunction: A New Analysis.* Washington, DC: The National Academies Press, 1994.

2. Pickering, L. K., ed., *Red Book: 2003 Report of the Committee on Infectious Diseases.* 26th ed. Elk Grove Village, IL: American Academy of Pediatrics, 2003.

3. Cherry, J. D. "Why Do Pertussis Vaccines Fail?" *Pediatrics* 129(5) (May 1, 2012):968–970.

4. Grens, K. "Whooping Cough Vaccine Fades in Pre-Teens: Study. Reuters, (Apr 3, 2012) http://www.reuters.com/article/2012/04/03/us-whoopingcough-idUSBRE8320 TM20120403 (accessed Oct 2012).

5. Pickering, L. K., ed., *Red Book: 2012 Report of the Committee on Infectious Diseases.* 29th ed. Elk Grove Village, IL: American Academy of Pediatrics, 2012.

6. Ibid.

7. Madsen, K. M., A. Hviid, M. Vestergaard, et al. "A Population-Based Study of Measles, Mumps, and Rubella Vaccination and Autism." *N Engl J Med* 347(19) (Nov 7, 2002):1477–82. Madsen, K. M., M. B. Lauritsen, C. B. Pedersen, et al. "Thimerosal and the Occurrence of Autism: Negative Ecological Evidence from Danish Population-Based Data." *Pediatrics* 112(3 Pt 1) (Sep 1,2003):604–606.

8. Adams, M. "CDC Vaccine Scientist Who Downplayed Links to Autism Indicted by DOJ in Alleged Fraud Scheme." Natural News.com, Apr 28, 2011. http://www.naturalnews.com/032216_Thorsen_fraud.html (accessed Oct 2012). Huff, E. A. "Exposed: CDC Deliberately Manipulated, Covered Up Scientific Data Showing Links Between Vaccines Containing Mercury and Autism." Natural News.com, Nov 2, 2011. http://www.naturalnews.com/034038_vaccines_autism.html (accessed Oct 2012).

Chapter 5. Feeding the Infant and Related Problems

1. Picciano, M. "Nutrient composition of human milk." *Pediatr Clin North Am* 48(1) (Feb 2001):53–67.

2. Berman, R. E., V. C. Vaughan, W. E. Nelson. *Nelson Textbook of Pediatrics*. Philadelphia: Saunders, 1987.

3. Blasbalg, T. L., J. R. Hibbeln, C. E. Ramsden, et al. "Changes in Consumption of Omega-3 and Omega-6 Fatty Acids in the United States During the 20th Century." *Am J Clin Nut* 93(5) (May 2011):950–962.

4. Journey to Crunchville, "Breastmilk Can Not Be Imitated—The DHA/ARA Fallout and Oligosaccharides," May 21, 2008. https://journeytocrunchville.wordpress.com/2008/05/21/breastmilk-can-not-be-imitated-the-dhaara-fallout-and-oligosaccharides/ (accessed October 23, 2012).

5. Holick, Michael F, et al. "Endocrine Society Issues Practice Guideline on Vitamin D." *Endocrine Soc 93rd Ann Meeting* (Jun 7, 2011).

6. Tromp, I. I., J. C. Kiefte-de Jong, A. Lebron, et al. "The Introduction of Allergenic Foods and the Development of Reported Wheezing and Eczema in Childhood."*Arch Pediatr Adolesc Med* 165(10) (Oct 2011):933–938.

7. Lino, M. *Expenditures on Children by Families, 2002*. USDA Center for Nutrition Policy and Promotion. Washington, DC, May 2003. Miscellaneous Publication Number 1528–2002. http://www.usda.gov/cnpp/Crc/crc2002.pdf (accessed Oct 2012).

Chapter 6. Well-Baby (and Child) Checkups

1. Hafton, N., G. D. Stevens, K. Larson, et al. "Duration of a Well-Child Visit: Association with Content, Family-Centeredness, and Satisfaction." *Pediatrics* 128(4) (Oct 1, 2011):657–664.

Chapter 7. Middle Ear Infections and Other Related Problems

1. National Institutes of Health. National Institute on Deafness and Other Communication Disorders. "Ear Infections in Children." NIH Publication No. 10–4799. http://www.nidcd.nih.gov/health/hearing/pages/earinfections.aspx (accessed Oct 2012).

Chapter 8. Colds, Influenza, and Other Respiratory Illnesses

1. FDA. U.S. Food and Drug Administration. "An Important FDA Reminder for Parents: Do Not Give Infants Cough and Cold Products Designed for Older Children." (Aug 3, 2011) http://www.fda.gov/Drugs/ResourcesForYou/SpecialFeatures/ucm263948.htm) (accessed Nov 2012).

Chapter 9. Fever: Its Significance and Management

1. Orlowski, J. P., J. Gillis, H. A. Kilhaun. "A Catch in the Reye." *Pediatrics* 80(5) (Nov 1987):638–642.

2. Pinsky, P. F., E. S. Hurwitz, L. B. Schonberger, et al. "Reye's Syndrome and Aspirin: Evidence for a Dose-Response Effect." *J Amer Med Assoc* 260(5) (Aug 5, 1988):657–661.

3. Khashab, M., A. J. Tector, P. Y. Kwo. "Epidemiology of Acute Live Failure." *Curr Gastroenterol Rep* 9(1) (Mar 9, 2007):66–73.

4. Little, J. A. "Acetaminophen and Reye's Syndrome?" *Pediatrics* 58(6) (Dec 1976):918.

5. Orlowski, J. P., J. Gillis, H. A. Kilhaun. "A Catch in the Reye." *Pediatrics* 80(5) (Nov 1987):638–642.

Chapter 10. Allergies

1. Ownby, D. R., C. C. Johnson, E. L. Peterson, ""Exposure to Dogs and Cats in the First Year of Life and Risk of Allergic Sensitization at 6 to 7 Years of Age" *J Amer Med Assn* 288(8) Aug 28, 2002):963–972.

Chapter 11. Over-the-Counter (OTC) Drugs

1. Hendeles, L. R. C. Hatton. "Oral Phenylephrine: An Ineffective Replacement for Pseudoephedrine?" *J Allergy Clin Immun* (letter) 118(1) (Jul 2006): 279–280].

2. Craig, D. G. C. M. Bates, J. S. Davidson, et al. "Staggered Overdose Pattern and Delay to Hospital Presentation are Associated with Adverse Outcomes Following Paracetamol-Induced Hepatotoxicity." *Brit J Clin Pharmaco* 73(2) (Feb 2012): 285–294.

Chapter 12. Child Rearing

1. Dobson, J. *The Strong-Willed Child*. Living Books, 1992.

Chapter 13. Sudden Infant Death Syndrome (SIDS)

1. Kalokerinos, A. *Medical Pioneer of the 20th Century: Dr. Archie Kalokerinos: An Autobiography*. NSW, Australia: Biological Therapies Publishing, 2000.

2. Follis, R. H. "Sudden Death In Infants With Scurvy." *J Pediatrics* (1942). http://www.whale.to/v/c/follis.html (accessed April 2013). Hattersley, J. G. "The Answer to Crib Death 'Sudden Infant Death Syndrome' (SIDS)" *J Orthomolecular Med* 1993. http://orthomolecular.org/library/jom/1993/pdf/1993-v08n04-p229.pdf (accessed April 2013).

Chapter 14. High-Dose Vitamin C Therapy for Young Children

1. For a discussion of bowel tolerance as an indicator of vitamin C saturation:

Cathcart, R. F. "Vitamin C, Titrating to Bowel Tolerance, Anascorbemia, and Acute Induced Scurvy." *Med Hypotheses* 7 (1981): 1359–1376. http://www.doctoryourself .com/titration.html (accessed Nov 2012). Cathcart, R. F. "The Third Face of Vitamin C." *J Orthomolecular Med* 7(4) (1993):197–200. http://www.doctoryourself.com/cath-cart_thirdface.html (accessed Nov 2012).

2. For more about Dr. Klenner's life and work: Saul, A. W. "Hidden in Plain Sight: The Pioneering Work of Frederick Robert Klenner, M.D." *J Orthomolecular Med* 22(1) (2007):31–38. http://www.doctoryourself.com/klennerbio.html (accessed Nov 2012).

3. Klenner, F. R. "The Significance of High Daily Intake of Ascorbic Acid in Preventive Medicine." in Williams, R. J., D. K. Kalita, editors. *A Physician's Handbook on Ortho-molecular Medicine.* 3rd ed. New York: Pergamon Press, 1977:51–59.

4. Hickey, S., H. Roberts. *Ascorbate: The Science of Vitamin C.* Morrisville, NC: Lulu, 2004.

5. Saul, A. W. "Vitamin C Has Been Known to Cure over 30 Major Diseases for over 50 Years." DoctorYourself.com. http://www.doctoryourself.com/vitaminc.html (accessed Nov 2012).

6. U.S. Department of Agriculture. "Animal Care Resource Guide, Dealer Inspection Guide. Animal Care. 12.4.2." http://www.aphis.usda.gov/animal_welfare/downloads/manuals/dealer/feeding.pdf (accessed Nov 2012).

7. Centers for Disease Control and Prevention. National Center for Health Statistics. "Americans Slightly Taller, Much Heavier than Four Decades Ago." (Oct 27, 2004). http://www.cdc.gov/nchs/pressroom/04news/americans.htm (accessed Nov 2012).

8. Saul, A. W. "Hidden in Plain Sight: The Pioneering Work of Frederick Robert Klen-ner, M.D." *J Orthomolecular Med* 22(1) (2007):31–38. http://www.doctor yourself.com/klennerbio.html (accessed Nov 2012).

9. Cathcart, R. F. "Delay by Intellectualization." http://www.orthomed.com. See also: http://orthomolecular.org/hof/2008/cathcart.html; http://www.doctoryourself.com/titration.html and http://www.doctoryourself.com/biblio_cathcart.html (accessed Nov 2012).

10. Bronstein, A.C., D. A. Spyker, L. R. Cantilena, et al. "2008 Annual Report of the American Association of Poison Control Centers' National Poison Data System (NPDS): 26th Annual Report." *Clin Toxicol* 47(10) (Dec 2009):911–1084. The full text article is available for free download at https://aapcc.s3.amazonaws.com/pdfs/annual_reports/NPDS_Annual_Report_2008_1.pdf. Vitamins statistics are found in Table 22B, journal pages 1052–3. Minerals, herbs, amino acids and other supplements are in the same table, pages 1047–8. Download any Annual Report of the American Association of Poison Control Centers from 1983–2008 free of charge at http://www.aapcc.org/annual-reports/ (accessed Nov 2012).

11. BMJ Publishing Group. *Clinical Evidence.* http://clinicalevidence.bmj.com/x/index.html (accessed Nov 2012).

12. 5. Morgan, G., R. Ward, M. Barton. "The Contribution of Cytotoxic Chemother-apy to 5-Year Survival in Adult Malignancies." *Clin Oncol (R Coll Radiol)* 16(8) (Dec 2004):549–560.

13. "Robert F. Cathcart, M.D. Key Articles, 1975–2005." http://www.doctoryourself.com/biblio_cathcart.html (accessed Nov 2012).

14. Stone, I. *The Healing Factor: "Vitamin C" against Disease.* New York: Grosset & Dunlap, 1974. The complete text of Irwin Stone's book *The Healing Factor* is posted for free reading at http://vitamincfoundation.org/stone/ (accessed Nov 2012).

15. Pauling, L. *How to Live Longer and Feel Better,* revised edition. Corvallis, OR: Oregon State Univ. Press, 2006.

16. Smith, L. H. *Clinical Guide to the Use of Vitamin C: The Clinical Experiences of Frederick R. Klenner, M.D.* Portland, OR: Life Sciences Press, 1988. Adapted from: *Vitamin C as a Fundamental Medicine: Abstracts of Dr. Frederick R. Klenner, M.D.'s Published and Unpublished Work.* Reprinted 1991. Available online at http://www.whale.to/a/smith_b.html (accessed April 2013).

17. Levy, T. E. *Vitamin C, Infectious Diseases, and Toxins: Curing the Incurable.* Philadelphia, PA: Xlibris Corporation, 2002.

Chapter 15. Environmental Hazards Affecting Infants and Toddlers

1. Trasande, L., T. M. Attina, J. Blustein. "Association Between Urinary Bisphenol A Concentration and obesity Prevalence in Children and Adolescents." *J Am Med Assn* 308(11) (Sep 19, 2012):1113–1121.

2. Swan, S. H., F. Liu, M. Hines, et al. "Prenatal Phthalate Exposure and Reduced Masculine Play in Boys." *Int J Androl* 33(2) (Apr 2010):259–69.

3. Swan, S. H., F. Liu, M. Hines, et al. "Sex-Typical Play Behavior in Boys May be Feminized by Maternal Exposure to Phthalates During Pregnancy" *Int J Androl* 32 (Nov 11, 2009):1–9.

4. Grandjean, P., E. W. Anderson, E. Budtz-Jørgensen, et al. "Serum Vaccine Antibody Concentrations in Children Exposed to Perfluorinated Compounds." *J Amer Med Assn* 307(4) (2012):391–397.

5. Nelson, R. "President's Cancer Panel: Environmental Cancer Risk Underestimated." Medscape Today News. May 13, 2010. http://www.medscape.com/viewarticle/721766 (accessed Nov 2012).

Chapter 16. Dispensing with Fluoride

1. American Association of Pediatrics. *Pediatric Nutrition Handbook.* Elk Grove Village, IL: American Academy of Pediatrics, 1985.

2. Ibid.

3. Fluoride Recommendations Work Group, CDC. "Recommendations for using fluoride to prevent and control dental caries in the United States." *MMWR Recommendations and Reports.* 50(RR14) (Aug 17, 2001):1–42. http://www.cdc.gov/mmwr/preview/mmwrhtml/rr5014a1.htm (accessed Nov 2012).

4. Saul., A. W. "How to Fool All of the People All of the Time. Orthomolecular.org http://www.orthomolecular.org/resources/omns/v06n05.shtml (accessed Nov 2012).

5. Peckham, S. "Slaying Sacred Cows: Is It Time to Pull the Plug on Water Fluoridation?" *Critical Public Health* 22(2) (2012):159–177. For an abstract of this report, scroll down at: http://www.fluorideresearch.org/444/files/FJ2011_v44_n4_p260–261 _sfs.pdf. This revised article originally appeared in Fluoride 2011, 44(4)188–190. It is reprinted with kind permission of the International Society for Fluoride Research Inc. www.fluorideresearch.org or www.fluorideresearch.com. Editorial Office: 727 Brighton Road, Ocean View, Dunedin 9035, New Zealand.

6. Hileman, B. "Fluoridation of Water: Questions About Health Risks and Benefits Remain after More Than 40 Years." *Chem Eng News* (American Chemical Society) 66(31) (Aug 1, 1988):26–42.

7. Foster, H.D. "Fluoride and Its Antagonists: Implications for Human Health." *J Orthomolecular Med* 8(3) (1993):149–153. http://orthomolecular.org/library/jom/1993/pdf/1993-v08n03-p149.pdf (accessed Nov 2012).

8. Meiers, P. "Does Water Fluoridation Have Negative Side Effects? A Critique of the York Review, Objective 4, Sections 9.1–9.6." *J Orthomolecular Med* 16(2) 2001): 73–82. http://www.orthomolecular.org/library/jom/2001/pdf/2001-v16n02-p073.pdf (accessed Nov 2012).

9. Yiamouyiannis, J. A. "Water Fluoridation and Tooth Decay: Results from the 1986–1987 National Survey of U.S. Schoolchildren." *Fluoride* 23(2) (Apr 1990):55–67. http://www.fluorideresearch.org/232/files/FJ1990_v23_n2_p055–067.pdf (accessed Nov 2012).

10. Hoffer, A. "More on Fluoride, Mercury and Teeth." editorial. *J Orthomolecular Med* 5(4) (1990):187–188. www.orthomolecular.org/library/jom/1990/pdf/1990-v05n04-p187.pdf (accessed Nov 2012). See also: Hileman, B. "New Studies Cast Doubt on Fluoridation Benefits." *Chem Eng News* SLweb.org (May 8, 1989). http://www.slweb.org/NIDR.html (accessed Nov 2012).

INDEX

ABOUT THE AUTHORS

Ralph K. Campbell, M.D., is a life-long advocate of nutritional medicine. He maintained a large private pediatric practice in Southern California for thirteen years and transitioned to Polson, Montana in 1970. He conducted well-child clinics for the Salish Kootenai reservation, established the Lake County Health Department, had a private pediatric practice, and served as a County jail doctor for thirteen years. His wide experience continues to invigorate his steady commitment to nutritionally oriented medicine, which has strengthened throughout numerous cultural changes in the medical community, even when he has had to make a great many efforts to buck the system.

Dr. Campbell grew up in Long Beach, California and married his high school sweetheart after graduating from Pomona College. He then moved to the East Coast to attend medical school at Yale University, where he received his M.D. degree in 1954. He completed his residency in pediatrics at Los Angeles Children's Hospital. He and his wife Jan also currently manage a commercial cherry orchard on Flathead Lake in Montana, which is greatly enjoyed by their five children and nine grandchildren.

Andrew W. Saul, Ph.D., has taught every grade there is, from first to post-doctoral, including nine years teaching for the State University of New York. He has published over 180 reviews and editorials in peer-reviewed publications. Dr. Saul is the author of *Doctor Yourself* and *Fire Your Doctor!*, and coauthor of *Orthomolecular Medicine for Everyone*; *The Vitamin Cure for Alcoholism*; *Vitamin C: The Real Story*; *I Have Cancer: What Should I Do?*; *Hospitals and Health*; *The Vitamin Cure for Depression*; *Vegetable Juicing for Everyone*; *Niacin: The Real Story* and, with Dr. Campbell, *The Vitamin Cure for Children's Health Problems*. All are available from Basic Health Publications.

Dr. Saul is on the editorial board of the *Journal of Orthomolecular Medicine*, is Editor-in-Chief of the *Orthomolecular Medicine News service*, and is featured in the documentary film *Food Matters*. In 2013, Dr. Saul was inducted into the Orthomolecular Medicine Hall of Fame. His noncommercial, natural-healing website is www.Doctor Yourself.com.

Most people's diets are woefully inadequate for providing proper nutrition. Even good diets fail to deliver sufficient levels of nutrients. The Vitamin Cure series highlights the safe and clinically effective use of vitamin supplements for a variety of illnesses. Research continues to prove the immense value of vitamins for maintaining health and fighting disease. The Vitamin Cure books, written by authors who are recognized experts in their field, offer authoritative, up-to-date, and practical information on taking vitamins for particular health problems.

THE VITAMIN CURE for Allergies
DAMIEN DOWNING

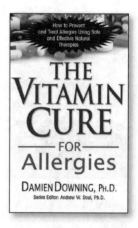

Throughout the developed world, the number of people with allergies—to inhalants, foods, and chemicals—has been rising for 50 years, and rising steeply for the last 20 years. Many allergy cases are misdiagnosed and people often don't find relief even when they are treated. The good news is that there are a number of commonsense steps you can take to relieve—and even prevent—allergies with *The Vitamin Cure for Allergies* as your guide:

- Avoid: Once you have discovered what sets you off, stay away from it. Remove anything to which you react, not only from your environment but from your body, too.

- Protect: Use nutrition—including vitamins C and D, essential fatty acids, and magnesium—to prevent or reduce allergy symptoms.

- Desensitize: Desensitization involves exposure to a small dose of an allergen in order to lessen your immune system's reaction. Options include homeopathic formulas, neutralization, and enzyme-potentiated desensitization (EPD).

Many people with allergies have experienced profound improvement by using the recommendations in this book. By incorporating these measures into your own life, you, too, can find lasting relief from allergies.

$14.95 • Trade Paperback • ISBN: 978-1-59120-271-4 • 144 Pages

THE VITAMIN CURE
for Alcoholism
ABRAM HOFFER & ANDREW W. SAUL

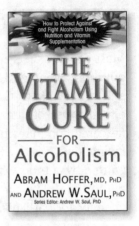

The Vitamin Cure for Alcoholism can help those who suffer from alcohol addiction, their friends and loved ones, and those in the relevant helping professions. Its central message is that alcoholism is primarily a metabolic disease that should be treated nutritionally first. The alcoholic suffers from nutrient deficiency, especially vitamin B3, and seeks relief by consuming alcohol. Megavitamin therapy is not only more effective than drugs or counseling, it is cheaper and safer. Behavioral and psychological treatments have lacked long-term success, largely because they pay little attention to the nutritional needs of alcoholics. In fact, Bill W., the man who cofounded Alcoholics Anonymous (AA), promoted the concept of megavitamin therapy. Nutrition can cure alcohol addiction.

$14.95 • Trade Paperback • ISBN: 978-1-59120-254-7 • 144 Pages

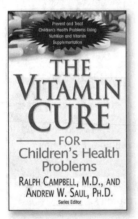

THE VITAMIN CURE
for Children's Health Problems
RALPH CAMPBELL & ANDREW W. SAUL

A healthy diet can have a profound impact on a child's development, helping him or her stay well and avoid illness. This is a practical guide to using therapeutic nutrition for common childhood illnesses that can be prevented and effectively treated with vitamins and other nutrients.

The Vitamin Cure for Children's Health Problems introduces readers to the concept of orthomolecular medicine to take control of their family's health. It covers pros and cons of antibiotics and vaccinations and looks at natural ways to boost immune function. Healthy eating for children is thoroughly covered, as are ways to protect children from a toxic environment. The book tackles three of the most pressing health issues for children: obesity and diabetes, allergies and asthma, and ADHD. It provides guidance on using therapeutic doses of vitamin C and other nutrients. The good news is that therapeutic nutrition is cheap, simple, effective, and safe.

$14.95 • Trade Paperback • ISBN: 978-1-59120-294-3 • 304 Pages

THE VITAMIN CURE
for Chronic Fatigue Syndrome
JONATHAN E. PROUSKY

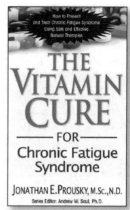

Chronic fatigue syndrome (CFS) is an elusive, difficult-to-treat condition in which the entire human organism has gone out of kilter. Symptoms include fatigue, muscle and joint pain, feeling unwell after exercise, unrefreshing sleep, and memory/concentration problems. Causes include allergies, nervous system dysfunction, environmental toxins, immune dysfunction, and oxidative stress.

This book directly addresses the causes of CFS and offers vitamin and other treatments capable of safely reducing symptoms. Orthomolecular therapy encompasses common vitamins in combination with sound medical and scientific evidence. These natural treatments can provide profound relief for those with chronic fatigue.

$14.95 • Trade Paperback • ISBN: 978-1-59120-268-4 • 160 Pages

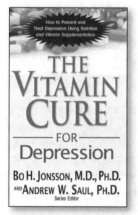

THE VITAMIN CURE
for Depression
BO H. JONSSON & ANDREW W. SAUL

This book reviews the multiple aspects that can be factors in depression, including the environmental, physical, and mental stresses of life. Many sufferers have never been encouraged or informed about nutritional medicine. *The Vitamin Cure for Depression* focuses on simple, safe, and easy nutritional treatments that anyone can try. Standard treatments ignore lifestyle and environmental factors such as food and toxins. The prognosis is often pessimistic and drug treatment is usually considered the best option.

Patients can certainly benefit from contact with a doctor, but should be involved in the important decisions regarding their treatment and aware of alternative or additional treatments. This book provides essential information on the benefits that vitamins, other nutrients, and lifestyle modifications can offer in an integrated treatment of depression. *The Vitamin Cure for Depression* offers a solid overview on depression and gives you the facts you need to help yourself feel better and stay healthier, both mentally and physically.

$14.95 • Trade Paperback • ISBN: 978-1-59120-282-0 • 240 Pages

THE VITAMIN CURE
for Diabetes
IAN E. BRIGHTHOPE

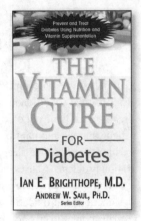

More than 220 million people worldwide have diabetes, and over 3 million people die from its consequences each year. Diabetes mellitus affects the use of sugar (glucose) in the body, either because the body does not produce enough insulin or the cells do not respond to it. High levels of blood glucose become toxic to tissues and organs and may cause blindness, kidney failure, brain and nerve damage, heart disease, and atherosclerosis.

The Vitamin Cure for Diabetes can help the majority of diabetics come off all or most medications by changing their lifestyle, eating a healthier diet, starting to exercise, and taking nutraceuticals. This book provides a complete supplement program (vitamins, minerals, and other dietary supplements) that can prevent or delay the onset of diabetes. Readers will learn how to optimally manage, or even prevent, diabetes for themselves and for their loved ones.

$14.95 • Trade Paperback • ISBN: 978-1-59120-290-5 • 208 Pages

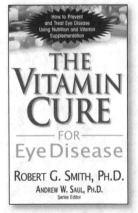

THE VITAMIN CURE
for Eye Disease
ROBERT G. SMITH

We often take our eyesight for granted until problems begin to develop. Many serious eye-related illnesses, from glaucoma to retinitis pigmentosa, are degenerative—they progress throughout our life and only reveal themselves later on. These age-related eye diseases, and many others, can be prevented or improved with proper nutrition and vitamin supplementation.

Robert Smith has written a comprehensive guidebook to aid in understanding the function of the eye and maintaining or regaining good eye health. *The Vitamin Cure for Eye Disease* introduces the complex workings of the eye and the illnesses that can occur through oxidative stress and poor nutrition. Dr. Smith guides us through the current research, explaining how correct vitamin supplementation and good nutrition can stave off or improve our visual health.

This book is indispensable for people seeking therapeutic, natural help for specific eye diseases and those wanting to maintain healthy eyes for life.

$14.95 • Trade Paperback • ISBN: 978-159120-292-9 • 208 Pages

THE VITAMIN CURE
for Heart Disease
HILLARY ROBERTS & STEVE HICKEY

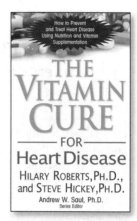

Heart disease is one of the main causes of death in the Western world—three in ten deaths are the result of cardiovascular disease, including heart attack, stroke, and aneurysm. Experts have often attributed cardiovascular disease primarily to "risk factors" such as high cholesterol. In fact, this does not even begin to tell the whole story.

The Vitamin Cure for Heart Disease examines the true causes of cardiovascular disease: inflammation and oxidation in the walls of arteries. Information on treatment and prevention focuses on safe alternatives to conventional drugs and surgery. This book shows readers how to stay heart healthy by making simple dietary changes, including reducing sugar intake; taking in adequate levels of B vitamins, as well as vitamins C and E; and supplementing the diet with fish oils.

Heart attack and stroke do not have to be an inevitable part of aging. Learn to take charge of your own heart health with safe and effective therapies.

$14.95 • Trade Paperback • ISBN: 978-1-59120-264-6 • 272 Pages

---

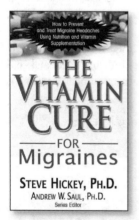

THE VITAMIN CURE
for Migraines
STEVE HICKEY

Migraine headaches are one of the most incapacitating diseases in terms of useful days lost. Worldwide, more than 300 million people are afflicted by migraines. Unfortunately, it is a chronic disease that is particularly difficult for conventional medicine to investigate or treat effectively.

Nutrition should be the first line of defense for a migraine sufferer. *The Vitamin Cure for Migraines* describes nutritional approaches to both prevention and treatment, based on orthomolecular (megavitamin) medicine. Additional noninvasive therapies that may be helpful include herbal medicine, acupuncture, and oxygen therapy. As a last resort, selected drugs can be used for aborting migraines—these are covered as well. With this safe and effective nutritional program, migraine sufferers' lives can be greatly improved.

$14.95 • Trade Paperback • ISBN: 978-1-59120-267-7 • 208 Pages

THE VITAMIN CURE
for Women's Health Problems
HELEN SAUL CASE

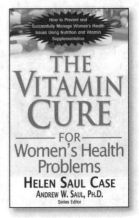

Women's health issues are often handled by physicians who have little time, and often no inclination, to get to the root cause of their patients' illnesses or concerns. Almost always, women are sent on their way after a quick diagnosis, with a prescription for what at first seems to be simple pharmaceutical answer to their problems.

Unfortunately medical solutions often don't work very well and have side effects that may seem as bad as or worse than the original illness. At best, they leave the person relying on drugs instead of addressing the root cause of the problem. Good nutritional guidance, natural alternative options, and vitamins that actually can cure are generally not options in the modern medical tool bag.

Helen Saul Case speaks from personal experience in dealing with her own health concerns in *The Vitamin Cure for Women's Health Problems*. She backs up her own knowledge of orthomolecular nutrition and its use for women's health issues with extensive research into the scientific studies of nutrition and supplementation, and she shares this information in an engaging, easy-to-read style.

This is a book all women will want to keep close by. It is a comforting reference resource for natural, drug-free alternatives to know about and consider for healthy everyday supplementation or when traditional medicine is not providing answers.

$18.95 • Trade Paperback • ISBN: 978-1-59120-274-5 • 304 Pages